SILENT KILLERS

UNVEILED

{PART 1}

EMPOWERING AWARENESS, PREVENTION, AND TREATMENT

BY

Peter Walker MD

Disclaimer

The information provided in this publication is for educational and informational purposes only. It does not constitute medical advice or substitute professional medical care. The author and publisher disclaim any liability for any adverse effects resulting from the use or application of the information contained herein. Readers should consult with a qualified healthcare professional for diagnosis, treatment, and personalized medical advice.

TABLE OF CONTENT

Silent Killers Unveiled.....................................1

{part 1} 1

Empowering Awareness, Prevention, and
Treatment 1

By 1

Introduction...9

The Concept of Silent Killers 9

Chapter 1 17

1.1 Understanding the Concept of Silent
Killers..17

1.2 The Importance of Early Detection and
Prevention 24

Chapter 2...33

Hypertension: The Silent Danger Lurking
Within 33

2.1 Exploring Hypertension and its Impact42

2.2 Risk Factors and Prevention Strategies51

1. Age:...52

2. Family history and genetics 52

3. Lifestyle factors 53

☐ Unhealthy diet......................................53

☐ Sedentary lifestyle: 54

☐ Tobacco and alcohol use 55

☐ Stress 55

☐ Adopting a healthy diet 57

☐ Engaging in regular physical activity 57

☐ Maintaining a healthy weight 58

☐ Limiting alcohol consumption: 59

☐ Quitting smoking: 59

☐ Managing stress 60

☐ Regular monitoring and check-ups 60

2.3 Treatment Options and Lifestyle Modifications 62

1. Lifestyle Adjustments: 63

2 . Medications: 67

Chapter 3 73

Diabetes: Silent Warfare on Our Body 73

1. Understanding Diabetes: 75

2. Impact of Diabetes on the Body: 77

3 . Managing Diabetes: 81

3.1 UNVEILING THE SILENT NATURE OF DIABETES 88

1. Subdued Symptoms: 90

2 . Possible Complications: 93

3 . Importance of Regular Screenings: 96

4 . Prevention and Management: 98
3.2 Types of Diabetes and their Effects ...102
1. Type 1 Diabetes: 103
Impacts: 104
2 . Type 2 Diabetes: 105
Impacts: 105
3 . Gestational Diabetes: 107
Impacts: 107
4 . Other Forms of Diabetes: 108
Impacts: 110
3.3 Managing Diabetes: Diet, Exercise, and
Medication 112
1. Diet: 113
2 . Exercise: 116
3 . Medication: 119
3.4 Complications and Long-Term Effects 123
1. Cardiovascular Complications: 124
2 . Nerve Damage (Neuropathy): 126
3 . KIDNEY DISEASE (NEPHROPATHY): 128
4 . Eye Complications: 130
5 . Foot Complications: 132
6 . Mental Health: 134
Chapter 4 137
Ovarian Cancer: The Whispering Threat . 137

Understanding Ovarian Cancer:...............139

Subtle Symptoms: 140

Risk Factors: 142

Early Detection and Prevention: 144

4.1 Understanding the Complexity and
Difficulties of Ovarian Cancer.................148

Different Types of Ovarian Cancer: 149

Challenges in Detection: 151

Challenges in Diagnosis:...........................153

Challenges in Treatment: 155

4.2 Risk Factors and Early Warning Signs158

Risk Factors: 159

Early Warning Signs:.................................162

Symptom Patterns: 163

Other Considerations: 164

Importance of Early Detection:.................165

4.3 Diagnosis and Treatment Options......167

Diagnosing Ovarian Cancer:.....................168

Staging Ovarian Cancer: 171

Treatment Options for Ovarian Cancer: ..173

Follow-up Care and Surveillance: 176

Clinical Trials: 177

4.4 Support and Assistance for Patients with
Ovarian Cancer 179

Support Groups: 180

Counseling and Mental Health Services:..181

Educational Resources:............................182

Fertility Preservation:..........................183

Financial and Practical Assistance:..........184

Palliative Care and Hospice Services: 185

Advocacy and Awareness Organizations:186

Personal Support Network: 187

Chapter 5 189

Colorectal Cancer: A Silent Journey to Danger....................................189

The Silent Progression of Colorectal Cancer:191

Risk Factors Associated with Colorectal 193

Screening and Early Detection: 195

Treatment Options for Colorectal Cancer:198

Prevention and Lifestyle Modifications:..202

5.1 The Stealthy Nature of Colorectal Cancer 206

Absence of Early Warning Signs:............207

Gradual Progression:.........................208

Non-specific Symptoms:..........................209

Importance of Tumor Location:...............210

Age and Genetic Factors:.........................211

Significance of Regular Screenings:........212

5.2 Screening and Detection Methods 214

Colonoscopy: 215

munochemical Test (FIT): 216

Fecal Occult Blood Test (FOBT):............217

Flexible Sigmoidoscopy: 218

Stool DNA Testing: 219

Virtual Colonoscopy (CT Colonography):220

5.3 Treatment Approaches and Survival

Rates...223

5.4 Promoting Awareness and Prevention231

Education and Information: 232

Screening Guidelines: 233

Risk Factor Awareness: 234

Lifestyle Modifications:........................235

Community Outreach and Engagement:..236

Survivor Stories and Support:................237

Chapter 6...239

Hepatitis C: Silent Liver Invader 239

The Hepatitis C Virus: 240

The Silent Nature of Hepatitis C:............241

Long-Term Effects and Complications:...242

Diagnosis and Testing:........................243

Treatment Options: 244

Prevention and Risk Reduction:............245

Public Health Efforts and Awareness: 246
Support and Care: 247
6.1 Unveiling Hepatitis C: Causes and
Transmission 249
The Hepatitis C Virus (HCV): 250
Transmission Modes: 251
Low-Risk Transmission Routes:..............254
Prevention: 255
6.2 Detecting Hepatitis C: Testing and
Diagnosis..260
Screening Recommendations:..................261
Antibody Testing: 262
Nucleic Acid Testing (NAT): 263
Genotype Testing:.................................264
Liver Function Tests: 264
Fibrosis Assessment:.............................265
Retesting and Monitoring: 266
Confidentiality and Support:....................267
6.3 Treatment Options and Management
Strategies...269
Antiviral Medications: 270
Monitoring and Follow-Up:......................272
Lifestyle Modifications:..........................273
Vaccination: 276

Emotional and Psychosocial Support: 277
Regular Liver Health Monitoring: 278
6.4 Education and Prevention Efforts 280
Raising Public Awareness: 281
Targeted Education: 282
Healthcare Provider Training:..................283
Screening and Testing Programs: 284
Harm Reduction Programs:.......................285
Prevention Strategies: 286
Collaboration and Partnerships:...............288
Access to Testing and Treatment:............289
Conclusion 291
Empowering Action against Silent Killersa291

INTRODUCTION

THE CONCEPT OF SILENT KILLERS

Within the realm of healthcare, there exists a group of diseases and conditions known as "silent killers," which pose a grave threat to our well-being. These insidious health risks have the ability to silently progress within our bodies, often without showing noticeable symptoms until they have reached an advanced stage. By the time their true nature is revealed, it may be too late for effective intervention. The concept of silent killers serves as a stark reminder of the significance of early detection, prevention, and proactive healthcare practices.

Silent killers encompass a variety of diseases and conditions, each with their own unique characteristics and potential consequences. Examples include hypertension (high blood pressure), diabetes, ovarian cancer, colorectal cancer, hepatitis C, atherosclerosis, and chronic kidney disease. What unifies them is their talent for disguising their presence, concealing themselves within the complexities of our bodies, and evading detection until intervention becomes challenging.

For instance, hypertension is appropriately named the "silent killer" because it often manifests without obvious symptoms. As blood pressure rises to dangerous levels, it silently causes damage to blood vessels, the heart, kidneys, and other organs, increasing the risk of severe complications such as heart disease, stroke, and kidney failure. Similarly, type 2 diabetes can develop inconspicuously, progressing over time without overt signs while silently causing disruption to blood sugar regulation, metabolism, and organ function.

Cancers also have the potential to emerge as silent killers. Ovarian cancer, characterized by its elusive symptoms and the absence of reliable screening methods, can grow undetected until it has spread to other parts of the body, complicating treatment. Colorectal cancer, another formidable silent killer, can remain symptomless for extended periods, only revealing itself at an advanced stage. Hepatitis C, a viral infection of the liver, silently leads to liver cirrhosis, liver cancer, and irreversible damage.

Atherosclerosis, the gradual buildup of plaque in arteries, silently progresses, narrowing blood vessels and heightening the risk of heart disease, heart attacks, and strokes. Chronic kidney disease can also quietly erode kidney function without obvious signs until it reaches an advanced stage, potentially leading to kidney failure necessitating dialysis or transplantation.

The covert nature of these silent killers highlights the importance of regular check-ups and screenings to detect these conditions early, when interventions are most effective. Consistent monitoring of blood pressure, blood glucose levels, and cancer screenings can aid in identifying potential issues before they become life-threatening.

Moreover, comprehending the risk factors associated with these conditions and adopting healthy lifestyle habits can play a crucial role in prevention. Maintaining a nutritious diet, engaging in regular exercise, managing stress, and abstaining from harmful behaviors such as smoking and excessive alcohol consumption can significantly reduce the risk of falling victim to these silent killers.

In this exploration of silent killers, we will delve into the specific characteristics of each condition, their potential consequences, and the available diagnostic and treatment options. By shedding light on these hidden dangers, our aim is to empower individuals to take control of their health by promoting awareness, early detection, and preventive measures. By exposing these stealthy adversaries, we can work towards a future where silent killers are defeated and lives are saved through proactive healthcare practices.

CHAPTER 1

1.1 UNDERSTANDING THE CONCEPT OF SILENT KILLERS

The notion of silent killers refers to diseases and conditions that can progress silently within the body, often without showing noticeable symptoms until they have already reached advanced stages. This poses a unique challenge for both healthcare professionals and individuals, as it requires

increased vigilance and proactive measures
to detect and address these hidden threats.
Silent killers defy our conventional
expectations of illness. We are accustomed
to associating diseases with evident
symptoms like pain, discomfort, or visible
signs of distress. However, silent killers
operate in a stealthy manner, quietly
undermining our health without being
detected.

There are several factors that contribute to
the phenomenon of silent killers. Firstly, the
human body is remarkably resilient and can
compensate for underlying issues, masking
symptoms until they become more severe.

This compensatory mechanism can create a false sense of well-being, causing individuals to overlook subtle warning signs that would typically prompt seeking medical attention.

Secondly, the complex nature of our physiological systems allows silent killers to develop discreetly. Diseases such as hypertension, diabetes, and atherosclerosis can progress slowly over a long period, subtly impairing vital functions without triggering obvious alarms. Sometimes, the body's adaptive mechanisms try to maintain balance despite underlying problems, further concealing the presence of a dangerous condition.

Thirdly, the lack of specific and recognizable symptoms adds to the silent nature of these diseases. Many silent killers manifest with vague or nonspecific signs that can easily be attributed to other causes or dismissed as unimportant. This further delays diagnosis and intervention, allowing the condition to advance unchecked.

Additionally, social and cultural factors contribute to perpetuating the silent killer phenomenon. Stigma, fear, and a lack of awareness surrounding certain diseases may discourage individuals from seeking medical attention or openly discussing their symptoms. This leads to delayed diagnosis and missed opportunities for early intervention.

To effectively combat the silent killer phenomenon, it is crucial to bring about a shift in healthcare practices. This involves promoting proactive healthcare measures, emphasizing regular check-ups, and advocating for comprehensive screenings. Healthcare providers should educate individuals about the importance of preventive care and empower them to take control of their health.

Public health initiatives aimed at raising awareness about silent killers and their associated risk factors can also have a significant impact. By educating communities about the subtle signs and symptoms, individuals can become more attuned to their bodies and recognize potential warning signs, prompting timely medical evaluation.

Furthermore, advancements in medical technology and diagnostic tools have the potential to improve the early detection of silent killers. Screening tests, genetic profiling, and imaging techniques allow for the identification of disease processes in their early stages, even before symptoms appear. This early detection enables healthcare professionals to intervene promptly and implement effective strategies to manage or treat the condition.

Understanding the concept of silent killers is crucial for addressing these hidden threats to our health. By acknowledging the complex interplay of physiological, social, and cultural factors, we can develop strategies to overcome the challenges posed by these elusive diseases. Through increased awareness, proactive healthcare practices, and advancements in diagnostics, we can unravel the phenomenon of silent killers and pave the way for early detection, prevention, and improved outcomes for individuals at risk.

1.2 THE IMPORTANCE OF EARLY DETECTION AND PREVENTION

The significance of early identification and prevention cannot be overstated when it comes to diseases that often go unnoticed. The saying "prevention is better than cure" holds true in this context, as timely detection and prevention play crucial roles in reducing the impact of these hidden ailments and enhancing overall health outcomes. By proactively recognizing and addressing such diseases in their early stages, individuals and healthcare systems can take vital steps to minimize the devastating consequences that can occur if left untreated.

Early detection is particularly important because many of these silent killers, including hypertension, diabetes, and certain forms of cancer, tend to progress gradually. They slowly undermine the body's normal functions and cause increasing damage over time. By detecting these conditions early, medical interventions can be initiated promptly, with the aim of slowing down or stopping their advancement.

Early detection allows healthcare professionals to intervene at a stage when treatment options are more effective. For instance, in the case of cancer, identifying malignancies during their initial phases often provides a wider range of treatment possibilities, such as less invasive surgeries, targeted therapies, or a higher chance of complete remission. Similarly, for conditions like hypertension and diabetes, early intervention through lifestyle changes, medications, and monitoring can help prevent or delay the onset of severe complications.

Furthermore, early detection can significantly improve the prognosis and overall survival rates for individuals affected by silent killers. Detecting diseases like ovarian cancer or colorectal cancer at an early stage, when they are confined to a specific area and haven't spread to distant sites, greatly increases the chances of successful treatment and long-term survival. Conversely, when these diseases are diagnosed in advanced stages, treatment options become more limited, and the prognosis becomes less favorable.

Prevention is equally essential in combating silent killers. Implementing preventive measures can help individuals reduce their risk of developing these diseases or identify them at an early stage. Prevention includes making lifestyle modifications such as maintaining a healthy diet, engaging in regular physical activity, and avoiding tobacco and excessive alcohol consumption. These measures have been proven to decrease the risk of developing conditions like hypertension, diabetes, and certain types of cancer.

Regular health check-ups and screenings also play a crucial role in prevention. Routine screenings, such as measuring blood pressure, testing blood glucose levels, conducting mammograms, colonoscopies, and pap smears, allow healthcare professionals to identify potential issues before symptoms manifest. These screenings can detect silent killers at their earliest stages, enabling prompt interventions.

Education and awareness campaigns are vital in fostering a proactive approach to health. By disseminating information about the risk factors, symptoms, and available preventive measures for silent killers, individuals can make informed choices and take steps to protect their health. Public health initiatives aimed at raising awareness about the importance of early detection and prevention can empower communities to prioritize regular screenings and adopt healthy lifestyles.

From a healthcare system perspective, emphasizing early detection and prevention can lead to significant benefits in terms of cost savings and resource allocation. Detecting diseases early reduces the need for extensive and costly treatments associated with advanced stages. Moreover, preventive measures and early interventions can help reduce the burden on healthcare systems by minimizing hospitalizations, emergency room visits, and long-term care needs.

Therefore early detection and prevention are crucial in combating silent killers that pose a substantial threat to our health. By identifying these diseases at their earliest stages, healthcare professionals can intervene promptly, improving treatment outcomes and survival rates. Emphasizing preventive measures, such as lifestyle modifications and regular screenings, empowers individuals to take control of their health and reduce their risk of developing these hidden conditions. Ultimately, a proactive approach to early detection and prevention is a powerful strategy to minimize the impact of silent killers and promote healthier lives.

CHAPTER 2

HYPERTENSION: THE SILENT DANGER LURKING WITHIN

Hypertension, also known as high blood pressure, is often referred to as the "silent killer" because it can progress unnoticed in the body. This stealthy condition affects millions of people globally and poses a significant risk to cardiovascular health. Understanding the nature of hypertension, its impact on the body, and the importance of detection and management are vital in preventing potential complications.

Essentially, hypertension is a chronic medical condition characterized by elevated blood pressure levels. Blood pressure represents the force exerted by circulating blood against the walls of blood vessels. While temporary increases in blood pressure are normal during physical exertion or stress, persistent high blood pressure can strain the cardiovascular system and lead to severe health issues.

The silent aspect of hypertension lies in its absence of apparent symptoms. Most individuals with high blood pressure do not experience noticeable signs until it reaches advanced stages or causes complications. Therefore, regular monitoring of blood pressure and medical check-ups are crucial for early detection.

Over time, untreated hypertension can have harmful effects on various organs and systems in the body. The constant pressure on the arterial walls can cause damage and contribute to the development of atherosclerosis, a condition characterized by the accumulation of plaque in the arteries.

This plaque buildup narrows the arteries, restricting blood flow and increasing the risk of cardiovascular events such as heart attacks and strokes.

Hypertension also places a significant burden on the heart. The heart has to work harder to pump blood against the increased resistance in the arteries, resulting in the enlargement of the heart muscle, known as hypertrophy. This can weaken the heart over time and contribute to the development of heart failure, a condition in which the heart is unable to pump blood effectively.

Additionally, high blood pressure can damage the kidneys, impairing their ability to filter waste products and maintain proper fluid and electrolyte balance in the body. Uncontrolled hypertension can lead to chronic kidney disease, further exacerbating the risk of complications.

Various factors contribute to the development of hypertension, including genetics, lifestyle choices, and underlying medical conditions. Risk factors such as a sedentary lifestyle, unhealthy eating habits (high sodium intake, low potassium intake), obesity, tobacco use, excessive alcohol consumption, and chronic stress can increase

the likelihood of developing hypertension.
Moreover, certain medical conditions like
diabetes, kidney disease, and sleep apnea
can contribute to the onset of high blood
pressure.

Managing hypertension requires a
comprehensive approach that often includes
lifestyle modifications and, in some cases,
medication. Lifestyle changes may involve
adopting a heart-healthy diet, engaging in
regular physical activity, maintaining a
healthy weight, limiting sodium intake,
moderating alcohol consumption, and
managing stress. Medications may be

prescribed to help lower blood pressure and effectively control the condition.

Regular blood pressure monitoring is crucial for detecting hypertension and assessing the effectiveness of treatment. Individuals with hypertension should work closely with healthcare professionals to establish a personalized management plan that includes regular check-ups, monitoring, and adjustments in lifestyle and medication as necessary.

Prevention plays a vital role in combating hypertension. By adopting healthy lifestyle habits from an early age, individuals can reduce their risk of developing high blood pressure. Public health initiatives, educational campaigns, and community programs that raise awareness about hypertension and its prevention can significantly contribute to reducing its prevalence.

Hypertension is rightly labeled as the silent danger lurking within. Its inconspicuous nature underscores the importance of proactive blood pressure monitoring, lifestyle modifications, and appropriate medical care. By increasing awareness, early detection, and effective management, individuals can mitigate the risks associated with hypertension and lead healthier lives.

2.1 EXPLORING HYPERTENSION AND ITS IMPACT

Hypertension, or high blood pressure, is a widespread medical condition that has a significant impact on individuals worldwide. It is characterized by consistently elevated levels of blood pressure, which places additional strain on the cardiovascular system. In this section, we will delve deeper into the specifics of hypertension, its effects on the body, and the potential risks if left unmanaged.

Blood pressure is measured in millimeters of mercury (mmHg) and is represented by two numbers: systolic pressure over diastolic pressure. Systolic pressure reflects the force exerted on arterial walls when the heart contracts, while diastolic pressure indicates the force between heartbeats when the heart is at rest. Normal blood pressure typically falls around 120/80 mmHg.

Hypertension is diagnosed when blood pressure consistently exceeds 130/80 mmHg. It is divided into two categories: primary (essential) hypertension and secondary hypertension. Primary hypertension accounts for the majority of cases and tends to develop gradually over time, influenced by a combination of genetic, lifestyle, and environmental factors. On the other hand, secondary hypertension is caused by an underlying medical condition, such as kidney disease, hormonal disorders, or certain medications.

The impact of hypertension on the body is multifaceted. Over time, the sustained high blood pressure can cause damage to the delicate inner lining of blood vessels, leading to the formation of plaque and narrowing of the arteries. This condition, known as atherosclerosis, restricts blood flow and can result in various complications.

One of the primary concerns with hypertension is its effect on the heart. The increased workload on the heart due to pumping blood against high resistance can lead to cardiac hypertrophy, which is the enlargement of the heart muscle. This hypertrophy may compromise the heart's ability to efficiently pump blood, potentially resulting in heart failure, a condition where the heart cannot meet the body's demands for blood and oxygen.

Hypertension is also a significant risk factor for cardiovascular events, including heart attacks and strokes. The narrowed arteries associated with atherosclerosis can become completely blocked or develop blood clots, depriving vital organs of oxygen and nutrients. This can lead to a heart attack if the blood supply to the heart is compromised or a stroke if blood flow to the brain is disrupted.

Furthermore, uncontrolled hypertension can adversely affect the kidneys, leading to chronic kidney disease. The high pressure within the blood vessels of the kidneys can damage their delicate filtering units (nephrons) and impair their ability to remove waste products and maintain proper fluid and electrolyte balance. In severe cases, chronic kidney disease can progress to end-stage renal disease, requiring dialysis or a kidney transplant.

The impact of hypertension extends beyond the cardiovascular system. It can also contribute to the development or worsening of other health conditions. For example, hypertension increases the risk of developing type 2 diabetes, a metabolic disorder characterized by high blood sugar levels. Additionally, hypertension can exacerbate existing eye conditions and contribute to vision loss.

Recognizing that hypertension is a chronic condition that often requires long-term management is crucial. Lifestyle modifications play a vital role in managing blood pressure. These modifications may include adopting a well-balanced diet low in sodium, engaging in regular physical activity, maintaining a healthy weight, limiting alcohol consumption, and managing stress.

In some cases, medication may be necessary to control blood pressure. Various classes of antihypertensive medications are available, including diuretics, beta-blockers, ACE inhibitors, angiotensin II receptor blockers (ARBs), calcium channel blockers, and others. The choice of medication depends on factors such as the individual's overall health, age, and any co-existing medical conditions.

Hypertension significantly affects the body, impacting multiple organ systems and increasing the risk of cardiovascular complications. Recognizing the importance of blood pressure control, adopting a healthy lifestyle, and closely collaborating with healthcare professionals are crucial steps in effectively managing hypertension. By controlling blood pressure levels, individuals can reduce the risks associated with hypertension and enhance their overall health and well-being.

2.2 RISK FACTORS AND PREVENTION STRATEGIES

It is crucial to comprehend the factors that contribute to the risk of hypertension in order to detect and prevent it early on. While certain factors such as age and genetics are beyond our control, there are several risk factors that individuals can modify to decrease their chances of developing high blood pressure. In this section, we will explore the common risk factors associated with hypertension and effective strategies for prevention.

1. **AGE:**

The likelihood of developing hypertension increases as individuals get older. This is mainly due to the natural aging process, which leads to the hardening and narrowing of the arteries. However, hypertension is not limited to older adults and can affect people of all age groups, including children and adolescents.

2. **FAMILY HISTORY AND GENETICS:**

Individuals with a family history of hypertension have a higher risk of developing the condition themselves.

Genetic factors can influence blood pressure regulation and sensitivity to environmental triggers. Although genetics cannot be changed, being aware of a family history of hypertension can prompt individuals to take proactive steps to monitor and manage their blood pressure.

3. LIFESTYLE FACTORS:

- ***UNHEALTHY DIET:***

  Consuming a diet that is high in sodium (salt), saturated and trans fats, and cholesterol can contribute to hypertension. Additionally, a lack of fruits, vegetables, and whole grains in the diet can deprive the body of essential nutrients and increase the risk of high blood pressure.

• *SEDENTARY LIFESTYLE:*

Physical inactivity and a lack of regular exercise can lead to weight gain, muscle loss, and an increased risk of hypertension. Engaging in regular physical activity can help maintain a healthy weight, strengthen the cardiovascular system, and lower blood pressure.

- ## *TOBACCO AND ALCOHOL USE*:

Smoking and excessive alcohol consumption can raise blood pressure and damage blood vessels, increasing the risk of hypertension. Quitting smoking and moderating alcohol intake are important steps in reducing this risk.

- ## *STRESS*:

Chronic stress and an inability to effectively manage it can contribute to hypertension. Prolonged stress can trigger the release of hormones that constrict blood vessels and increase blood pressure. Implementing stress-reduction techniques, such as exercise, meditation, and relaxation techniques, can help mitigate the impact of stress on blood pressure.

4 OBESITY AND OVERWEIGHT:

Having excess body weight, particularly around the waist, increases the risk of developing hypertension. Obesity is associated with various metabolic changes, including insulin resistance and inflammation, which can disrupt normal blood pressure regulation.

To prevent hypertension and maintain optimal blood pressure levels, the following strategies are recommended:

- ***ADOPTING A HEALTHY DIET:***

Emphasize a diet that is rich in fruits, vegetables, whole grains, lean proteins, and low-fat dairy products. Limit the consumption of sodium (less than 2,300 mg per day) and reduce the intake of saturated and trans fats.

- ***ENGAGING IN REGULAR PHYSICAL ACTIVITY:***

Aim for at least 150 minutes of moderate-intensity aerobic exercise or 75 minutes of vigorous-intensity exercise per week. Additionally, include strength training exercises at least twice a week to improve overall cardiovascular health.

• *MAINTAINING A HEALTHY WEIGHT*:

Strive to achieve a body mass index (BMI) within the normal range ($18.5\text{-}24.9 \text{ kg/m}^2$). Losing weight if overweight or obese can significantly reduce the risk of developing hypertension.

• *LIMITING ALCOHOL CONSUMPTION:*

 For men, limit alcohol intake to two standard drinks per day, and for women, limit it to one standard drink per day. Excessive alcohol consumption can raise blood pressure and contribute to other health problems.

• *QUITTING SMOKING:*

If you are a smoker, quitting is crucial for overall health. Smoking damages blood vessels and increases the risk of hypertension and other cardiovascular diseases. Seek support from healthcare

professionals and smoking cessation
programs to help quit smoking.

• *MANAGING STRESS*:

Implement stress-reduction techniques such
as exercise, meditation, deep breathing
exercises, or engaging in hobbies and
activities that bring joy and relaxation.

• *REGULAR MONITORING AND CHECK-UPS*:

Measure and monitor blood pressure levels
regularly. Routine check-ups with healthcare
professionals can help detect any changes or

abnormalities early on and allow for timely intervention.

By addressing these risk factors and adopting a healthy lifestyle, individuals can significantly reduce their chances of developing hypertension and its associated complications. It is important to remember that prevention requires a lifelong commitment, and making small changes in daily habits can make a substantial difference in maintaining optimal blood pressure and overall cardiovascular health.

2.3 TREATMENT OPTIONS AND LIFESTYLE MODIFICATIONS

The management of hypertension often involves a combination of lifestyle changes and, in some instances, medication. The treatment plan can vary depending on factors such as an individual's blood pressure levels, overall health, and any underlying medical conditions. In this section, we will explore the commonly recommended treatment options and lifestyle modifications for individuals with hypertension.

1. LIFESTYLE ADJUSTMENTS:

- Dietary Modifications: A heart-healthy diet, such as the DASH (Dietary Approaches to Stop Hypertension) diet, can effectively lower blood pressure. This diet emphasizes consuming fruits, vegetables, whole grains, lean proteins, and low-fat dairy products, while limiting sodium, saturated fats, and cholesterol. It is particularly important for individuals with hypertension to reduce their sodium intake to less than 2,300 milligrams per day (or even lower for certain individuals).

- Regular Exercise: Engaging in regular
  aerobic exercises like brisk walking,
  cycling, or swimming can help lower
  blood pressure. It is recommended to aim
  for at least 150 minutes of moderate-
  intensity aerobic activity or 75 minutes of
  vigorous-intensity aerobic activity per
  week, along with muscle-strengthening
  activities at least twice a week.

- Weight Management: Maintaining a
  healthy weight through a balanced diet
  and regular exercise is crucial for
  managing hypertension. Losing excess
  weight can significantly reduce blood

pressure and alleviate strain on the cardiovascular system.

- Moderating Alcohol Consumption: Consuming excessive amounts of alcohol can raise blood pressure. It is advised to limit alcohol intake to moderate levels, which means no more than two standard drinks per day for men and one standard drink per day for women.

- Smoking Cessation: Quitting smoking is essential for overall cardiovascular health. Smoking damages blood vessels, increases blood pressure, and raises the risk of heart disease. Seeking support from healthcare professionals, smoking cessation programs, or support groups can be highly beneficial in quitting smoking.

- Stress Management: Chronic stress can contribute to high blood pressure. Implementing stress-reducing techniques like exercise, meditation, deep breathing exercises, or engaging in hobbies and activities that promote relaxation can help manage stress and improve blood pressure control.

2. MEDICATIONS:

- Diuretics: Diuretics help the kidneys eliminate excess sodium and water from the body, thereby reducing blood volume and lowering blood pressure. They are commonly prescribed as the first-line treatment for hypertension.

- Beta-blockers: Beta-blockers reduce heart rate and the force of heart contractions, easing the workload on the heart and lowering blood pressure. They are often prescribed for individuals with certain

heart conditions in addition to
hypertension.

- ACE inhibitors (Angiotensin-Converting
Enzyme inhibitors) and ARBs
(Angiotensin II Receptor Blockers):
These medications help relax and widen
blood vessels, making it easier for blood
to flow and reducing blood pressure.

- Calcium channel blockers: Calcium
channel blockers prevent calcium from
entering the muscle cells of the heart and
blood vessels, leading to relaxation of
blood vessels and decreased blood
pressure.

- Other Medications: In some cases, additional medications such as alpha-blockers, central-acting agents, or direct renin inhibitors may be prescribed to control blood pressure.

It is important to note that the choice of medications and their dosages may vary depending on an individual's specific needs and any other existing medical conditions. Regular follow-ups with healthcare professionals are necessary to monitor blood pressure levels, make adjustments to medications if necessary, and evaluate the overall effectiveness of the treatment plan.

The most effective management of hypertension is achieved by combining lifestyle modifications with medication. It is crucial to maintain open communication with healthcare professionals, follow their recommendations, and attend regular check-ups to ensure blood pressure is well-controlled.

In certain cases, individuals may require additional interventions such as procedures or surgeries to manage underlying conditions contributing to hypertension. These interventions are typically reserved for severe cases or when lifestyle modifications and medications alone are insufficient in achieving blood pressure control.

Remember, hypertension is a chronic condition that requires ongoing management. By implementing healthy lifestyle changes, adhering to prescribed medications, and receiving regular medical care, individuals can effectively control blood pressure, reduce the risks associated with hypertension, and improve overall cardiovascular health.

CHAPTER 3

DIABETES: SILENT WARFARE ON OUR BODY

Diabetes, a chronic metabolic disorder affecting millions worldwide, is often dubbed a "silent" disease due to its subtle or unnoticed symptoms. However, beneath its seemingly unobtrusive façade, diabetes wages an ongoing battle within our bodies, wreaking havoc on multiple organ systems and posing grave health risks. In this section, we will delve into the impact of diabetes and stress the importance of comprehending and effectively managing this covert warfare.

1. UNDERSTANDING DIABETES:

Diabetes mellitus is characterized by persistently high blood glucose levels, stemming from either insufficient insulin production (Type 1 diabetes) or the body's ineffective use of insulin (Type 2 diabetes). Insulin, a hormone produced by the pancreas, regulates glucose metabolism and facilitates the transfer of glucose from the bloodstream into cells for energy.

Type 1 diabetes arises when the immune system mistakenly attacks and destroys the insulin-producing cells in the pancreas, resulting in a complete absence of insulin. Typically diagnosed in childhood or adolescence, Type 1 diabetes requires lifelong insulin therapy.

In contrast, Type 2 diabetes is commonly associated with lifestyle factors and genetic predisposition. In this form of diabetes, the body becomes resistant to insulin or the pancreas gradually loses its ability to produce adequate amounts of insulin. Type 2 diabetes is more prevalent and can often be managed through a combination of lifestyle adjustments, oral medications, and, in some cases, insulin therapy.

2. IMPACT OF DIABETES ON THE BODY:

- Cardiovascular System: Diabetes significantly heightens the risk of developing cardiovascular diseases, including heart attacks, strokes, and peripheral vascular disease. Elevated blood glucose levels can inflict damage on blood vessels, leading to atherosclerosis (hardening and narrowing of the arteries), increased blood pressure, and an augmented risk of blood clots.

- Nervous System: Prolonged high blood glucose levels can cause nerve damage throughout the body, resulting in a condition known as diabetic neuropathy. Diabetic neuropathy commonly affects the feet and legs, causing pain, tingling, numbness, and diminished sensation. It can also affect the digestive system, leading to issues such as gastroparesis (delayed stomach emptying) and diabetic neuropathy of the bladder, causing urinary problems.

- Eyes: Diabetes can impair blood vessels in the retina, leading to a condition called diabetic retinopathy. Diabetic retinopathy is a leading cause of vision loss and blindness in adults. Additionally, diabetes increases the risk of developing other eye conditions, including cataracts and glaucoma.

- Kidneys: Prolonged high blood glucose levels and hypertension can harm the kidneys over time, resulting in diabetic nephropathy. Diabetic nephropathy is a progressive condition that can lead to kidney failure and necessitate dialysis or a kidney transplant.

- Feet: Diabetes can impede blood circulation and diminish sensation in the feet, elevating the risk of foot ulcers and infections. If left untreated, these complications can lead to severe infections and, in severe cases, amputation.

- Other Complications: Diabetes can also affect the reproductive system, increase the risk of gum disease, impede wound healing, and impair the body's immune response.

3 . MANAGING DIABETES:

- Although diabetes may engage in a silent conflict within our bodies, its detrimental effects can be mitigated through effective management. Proper diabetes management focuses on maintaining blood glucose levels within the target range and controlling other risk factors. Here are key strategies for managing diabetes:

- Blood Glucose Monitoring: Regularly monitoring blood glucose levels enables individuals to understand how their bodies respond to different foods, medications, and activities. This information empowers them to make necessary adjustments in their diet, medication, and lifestyle choices to maintain optimal blood glucose control.

- Medications: Depending on the type of diabetes and individual circumstances, medications may be prescribed to manage blood glucose levels. These can include insulin injections, oral medications that enhance insulin sensitivity or stimulate insulin production, and other medications to control associated conditions such as high blood pressure and high cholesterol.

- Healthy Eating: Adopting a balanced, nutrient-rich diet is crucial in managing diabetes. This involves consuming a variety of whole grains, lean proteins, healthy fats, and ample fruits and vegetables. Controlling portion sizes, limiting the intake of sugary and processed foods, and monitoring carbohydrate consumption are important strategies for regulating blood glucose levels.

- Regular Physical Activity: Engaging in regular physical activity improves insulin sensitivity, lowers blood glucose levels, helps with weight control, and strengthens the cardiovascular system. Striving for at least 150 minutes of moderate-intensity aerobic exercise, such as brisk walking or swimming, per week, along with strength training exercises, is recommended.

- Weight Management: Achieving and maintaining a healthy weight is beneficial for managing diabetes. Weight loss, if overweight, can significantly improve insulin sensitivity and blood glucose control.

- Medication Adherence: Adhering to prescribed medications as directed by healthcare professionals is crucial. Proper adherence to medication regimens helps maintain stable blood glucose levels and reduces the risk of complications.

- Regular Medical Care: Routine check-ups with healthcare professionals are essential for monitoring blood glucose levels, assessing overall health, and detecting early signs of complications. Regular eye exams, foot exams, and screenings for other diabetes-related conditions are also recommended.

- Diabetes Education and Support: Acquiring knowledge about diabetes, its management, and lifestyle modifications empowers individuals to make informed decisions and better manage their condition. Diabetes education programs and support groups provide valuable

information, resources, and emotional
support.

Diabetes may wage a hidden conflict within
our bodies, but we need not face this battle
alone. With proper understanding,
awareness, and effective management
strategies, individuals can minimize the
impact of diabetes and lead healthy,
fulfilling lives. By proactively managing
blood glucose levels, addressing risk factors,
and seeking support from healthcare
professionals, individuals can navigate the
challenges of diabetes and reduce the risks
of associated complications. Remember,
early detection, self-care, and ongoing

support are essential tools in the fight against diabetes.

3.1 UNVEILING THE SILENT NATURE OF DIABETES

Diabetes, often known as the "silent disease," possesses deceptive traits that can catch individuals off guard. Many people with diabetes remain unaware of their condition until symptoms or complications arise. The silent nature of diabetes underscores the importance of comprehending the disease and implementing regular screenings and preventive measures. In this section, we will delve deeper into the concealed features of diabetes and the implications they have for individuals and healthcare systems.

1. SUBDUED SYMPTOMS:

Diabetes often advances quietly, with individuals experiencing few noticeable symptoms, particularly in the early stages. This can result in delayed diagnosis and missed opportunities for early intervention. However, there are some common indicators that may suggest the presence of diabetes:

- Frequent urination: Increased urine production due to elevated blood glucose levels.
- Excessive thirst: Persistent thirst caused by dehydration resulting from frequent urination.

- Fatigue: Feeling tired and lacking energy, even with sufficient rest.

- Unexplained weight loss: Losing weight despite normal or increased appetite.

- Blurry vision: Fluctuations in blood sugar levels affecting the lens of the eye.

- Slow wound healing: Delayed healing of cuts, sores, or bruises.

- Recurrent infections: Increased susceptibility to infections, particularly in the urinary tract, skin, and gums.

It is important to note that these symptoms can be mild or easily attributed to other factors, leading to a lack of suspicion or urgency to seek medical attention. Therefore, regular screenings and awareness of risk factors are crucial for early detection.

2 . POSSIBLE COMPLICATIONS:

The silent nature of diabetes becomes particularly concerning when considering the potential long-term complications that can arise if the disease remains unmanaged. Prolonged elevated blood glucose levels can damage blood vessels and organs, giving rise to various complications:

- Cardiovascular disease: Diabetes significantly increases the risk of heart attacks, strokes, and peripheral vascular disease.
- Kidney disease: Diabetes is a leading cause of chronic kidney disease, which

may progress to end-stage renal disease requiring dialysis or transplantation.

- Nerve damage: Prolonged high blood glucose levels can damage nerves throughout the body, resulting in diabetic neuropathy. This condition can cause pain, numbness, tingling, and problems with digestion, sexual function, and coordination.

- Eye problems: Diabetes can cause damage to the blood vessels in the retina, leading to diabetic retinopathy, which can cause vision loss and blindness.

- Foot complications: Diabetes can impair blood circulation and nerve function in the feet, increasing the risk of foot ulcers, infections, and, in severe cases, amputation.

- Skin conditions: Uncontrolled diabetes can lead to various skin problems, including bacterial and fungal infections, itching, and slow wound healing.

These complications can significantly impact an individual's quality of life and may necessitate extensive medical interventions and ongoing management.

3 . IMPORTANCE OF REGULAR SCREENINGS:

Given the silent nature of diabetes, routine screenings play a crucial role in early detection and prevention of complications. Healthcare professionals often recommend the following screenings:

- Blood glucose testing: This involves measuring fasting blood sugar levels or performing an oral glucose tolerance test to assess how the body handles glucose.

- Hemoglobin A1C test: This test provides an average blood sugar level over the past two to three months, offering an indication of long-term blood glucose control.

- Lipid profile: Regular lipid profile testing is essential to monitor cholesterol levels, as individuals with diabetes are at a higher risk of developing cardiovascular disease.

These screenings are particularly important for individuals with risk factors such as obesity, a sedentary lifestyle, a family history of diabetes, or previous gestational diabetes.

4 . PREVENTION AND MANAGEMENT:

Although diabetes may possess a silent nature, proactive measures can be taken to prevent or effectively manage the disease:

- Lifestyle modifications: Adopting a healthy lifestyle that includes regular physical activity, a balanced diet rich in fruits, vegetables, whole grains, lean proteins, and healthy fats, as well as weight management, can significantly reduce the risk of developing diabetes.

- Medication and insulin therapy: For individuals with diabetes, adhering to prescribed medications, insulin therapy, or other recommended treatments is crucial for maintaining blood glucose control.

- Regular healthcare visits: Individuals with diabetes should schedule regular check-ups to monitor blood glucose levels, assess overall health, and identify any early signs of complications.

- Diabetes education and support: Acquiring knowledge about diabetes self-care, including blood sugar monitoring, medication management, healthy eating, and stress management, can empower individuals to actively manage their condition and reduce the risk of complications.

The quiet characteristics of diabetes underscore the need for awareness, regular screenings, and proactive management. By comprehending the potential risks and complications associated with diabetes, individuals can take steps to prevent the disease or effectively manage it. Healthcare systems also play a vital role in promoting diabetes education, ensuring access to screenings, and providing support for individuals with diabetes. Through early detection, preventive measures, and ongoing care, the silent nature of diabetes can be addressed, enabling individuals to lead healthier lives and reducing the burden on healthcare systems.

3.2 TYPES OF DIABETES AND THEIR EFFECTS

Diabetes is a complex metabolic condition that can manifest in various ways, each with its own distinct characteristics and effects on the body. A comprehensive understanding of the different types of diabetes is vital in determining suitable management strategies and ensuring the best possible health outcomes. In this section, we will explore the diverse types of diabetes and their impacts on individuals.

1. TYPE 1 DIABETES:

Type 1 diabetes, also known as insulin-dependent or juvenile-onset diabetes, is an autoimmune disorder in which the body's immune system erroneously attacks and destroys the insulin-producing cells in the pancreas. Consequently, individuals with type 1 diabetes have minimal to no insulin production, necessitating lifelong insulin therapy.

IMPACTS:

- Insulin reliance: People with type 1 diabetes depend on external insulin to regulate their blood glucose levels.

- Fluctuating blood sugar levels: Insufficient insulin hampers the effective entry of glucose into cells, resulting in elevated blood sugar levels.

- Heightened risk of complications: Poorly managed type 1 diabetes can give rise to a range of complications, including cardiovascular disease, kidney damage, nerve damage, and eye problems.

2 . TYPE 2 DIABETES:

Type 2 diabetes, the most common form of diabetes, typically develops later in life and is often associated with lifestyle factors such as an unhealthy diet, sedentary behavior, and obesity. In type 2 diabetes, the body becomes resistant to insulin's effects, or there is inadequate insulin production.

IMPACTS:

- Insulin resistance: Cells become less responsive to insulin, impairing glucose uptake and leading to elevated blood sugar levels.

- Progressive nature: Type 2 diabetes tends to worsen over time as insulin resistance increases and insulin production declines.

- Heightened risk factors: Type 2 diabetes is closely linked to obesity, high blood pressure, high cholesterol levels, and a sedentary lifestyle.

- Potential for lifestyle management: Unlike type 1 diabetes, type 2 diabetes can sometimes be managed through lifestyle changes like weight loss, healthy eating, regular exercise, and, if necessary, medication.

3 . GESTATIONAL DIABETES:

Gestational diabetes occurs during pregnancy when hormonal changes affect insulin function. It typically resolves after delivery, but women who have had gestational diabetes are at an increased risk of developing type 2 diabetes later in life.

IMPACTS:

- Increased risks for the mother and baby: Poorly controlled gestational diabetes can lead to complications during pregnancy and childbirth, such as preeclampsia, high birth weight, and the need for a cesarean delivery.

- Future risk: Women who have had gestational diabetes face a higher likelihood of developing type 2 diabetes in the future and should undergo regular screenings.

4 . OTHER FORMS OF DIABETES:

There are several other forms of diabetes, including:

- LADA (Latent Autoimmune Diabetes in Adults): LADA is a slowly progressing form of autoimmune diabetes that initially appears as type 2 diabetes but eventually necessitates insulin treatment.

- MODY (Maturity-Onset Diabetes of the Young): MODY is a rare genetic form of diabetes that typically manifests before the age of 25 and is caused by specific gene mutations.

- Secondary Diabetes: Certain medical conditions, medications, hormonal disorders, and pancreatic diseases can lead to secondary diabetes.

IMPACTS:

- Unique characteristics: These forms of diabetes exhibit specific features and require treatment approaches that differ from type 1 and type 2 diabetes.
- Individualized management: Diagnosis and treatment of these forms of diabetes

necessitate careful evaluation by healthcare professionals.

Comprehending the various types of diabetes is crucial for accurate diagnosis, appropriate treatment plans, and targeted management strategies. It enables healthcare professionals to tailor interventions and support individuals in achieving optimal blood sugar control, reducing the risk of complications, and improving overall health outcomes.

3.3 MANAGING DIABETES: DIET, EXERCISE, AND MEDICATION

Managing diabetes involves effectively controlling blood sugar levels, reducing the risk of complications, and improving overall health outcomes. The management approach varies depending on the type of diabetes and individual needs, but generally involves a combination of dietary changes, regular physical activity, and medication. This section explores the key components of diabetes management and their impact on blood sugar control.

1. DIET:

Diet plays a crucial role in managing diabetes by influencing blood sugar levels, body weight, and overall health. The main goals of a diabetes-friendly diet include:

- Carbohydrate management: Monitoring and controlling carbohydrate intake is essential as it has the greatest impact on blood sugar levels. Balancing carbohydrate intake with insulin or medication, opting for complex carbohydrates with a low glycemic index, and spacing out meals can help maintain stable blood sugar levels.

- Portion control: Controlling portion sizes is important to avoid excessive calorie intake, manage weight, and regulate blood sugar levels. Including balanced meals with appropriate portions of carbohydrates, proteins, and healthy fats is key.

- Balanced meals: Emphasizing a diet rich in fruits, vegetables, whole grains, lean proteins, and healthy fats provides essential nutrients, fiber, and antioxidants. It is recommended to limit or avoid sugary beverages, processed foods, and saturated fats.

- Glycemic index: Considering the glycemic index (GI) of foods helps manage blood sugar levels. Low GI foods cause a slower rise in blood sugar compared to high GI foods.

Individualized dietary recommendations should be developed with the assistance of a registered dietitian or healthcare professional to meet specific needs, preferences, and medical requirements.

2 . EXERCISE:

Regular physical activity is a cornerstone of diabetes management, regardless of the type of diabetes. Exercise offers numerous benefits, including:

- Improved insulin sensitivity: Physical activity enhances the body's ability to use insulin effectively, leading to better blood sugar control.

- Weight management: Exercise helps maintain a healthy weight or supports weight loss, reducing insulin resistance and improving metabolic health.

- Cardiovascular health: Engaging in aerobic activities such as walking, jogging, cycling, or swimming strengthens the heart, lowers blood pressure, and reduces the risk of cardiovascular complications associated with diabetes.

- Stress management: Exercise acts as a natural stress reliever, promoting mental well-being and potentially aiding in blood sugar regulation.

- Muscle strength and flexibility: Incorporating resistance training and flexibility exercises improves muscle strength, joint flexibility, and balance, which are essential for overall physical fitness.

It is advisable to consult with a healthcare professional before starting an exercise program to ensure safety and develop an individualized plan based on fitness level, medical history, and specific needs.

3 . MEDICATION:

Medication management is often necessary in diabetes management, particularly for individuals with type 1 diabetes, advanced type 2 diabetes, or other forms of diabetes. Common medications used include:

- Insulin: Insulin therapy is crucial for individuals with type 1 diabetes and may be necessary for some with type 2 diabetes. It helps regulate blood sugar levels by facilitating glucose uptake into cells.
- Oral medications: Various oral medications help control blood sugar

levels in individuals with type 2 diabetes. These medications work by increasing insulin production, improving insulin sensitivity, or reducing glucose production in the liver.

- Injectable medications: In addition to insulin, injectable medications such as GLP-1 receptor agonists and SGLT2 inhibitors may be prescribed to control blood sugar levels, promote weight loss, and reduce cardiovascular risk factors.

Medication management should always be overseen by a healthcare professional who can determine the most suitable medication regimen, monitor its effectiveness, and adjust dosages as needed.

It's important to note that diabetes management is personalized, and treatment plans may vary based on factors such as age, overall health, presence of complications, and personal preferences. Regular monitoring of blood sugar levels, routine healthcare visits, and open communication with healthcare professionals are crucial for successful diabetes management. By incorporating a healthy diet, regular exercise, and appropriate medication, individuals with diabetes can effectively manage their condition and lead fulfilling, healthy lives.

3.4 COMPLICATIONS AND LONG-TERM EFFECTS

Diabetes, a chronic condition, can have various complications and long-term effects if not properly controlled. Managing blood sugar levels alone is not enough, highlighting the importance of diligent disease management and proactive measures. In this section, we will explore the potential complications and long-term effects associated with diabetes.

1. CARDIOVASCULAR COMPLICATIONS:

Diabetes significantly raises the risk of developing cardiovascular diseases, including:

- Heart disease: People with diabetes are more prone to coronary artery disease, heart attacks, and chest pain (angina).
- Stroke: Diabetes can lead to the narrowing and hardening of blood vessels, increasing the risk of stroke.

- Peripheral arterial disease: Reduced blood flow to the limbs can result in poor wound healing, infections, and, in severe cases, amputation.

- High blood pressure: Diabetes contributes to elevated blood pressure levels, increasing the risk of heart disease and stroke.

- To reduce the risk of cardiovascular complications, it is crucial to manage diabetes by controlling blood sugar, engaging in regular exercise, following a healthy diet, and using medication when necessary.

2 . NERVE DAMAGE (NEUROPATHY):

Prolonged high blood sugar levels can damage nerves throughout the body, resulting in diabetic neuropathy. Different types of neuropathy associated with diabetes include:

- Peripheral neuropathy: This condition affects the peripheral nerves, leading to numbness, tingling, pain, and weakness in the extremities, usually starting in the feet and hands.

- Autonomic neuropathy: Damage to the nerves controlling involuntary bodily functions can result in digestive issues, sexual dysfunction, problems with bladder control, and cardiovascular abnormalities.

- Focal neuropathy: Specific nerves become damaged, leading to sudden weakness or pain in specific muscles or groups of muscles.

To prevent or slow down the progression of neuropathy, it is important to maintain stable blood sugar levels, practice regular foot care, and manage other risk factors like smoking and high blood pressure.

3. KIDNEY DISEASE (NEPHROPATHY):

Diabetes is a leading cause of chronic kidney disease. Over time, high blood sugar levels can damage the tiny blood vessels in the kidneys, impairing their function. Key considerations include:

- Diabetic nephropathy: Kidney damage caused by diabetes can result in protein leakage in the urine, high blood pressure, fluid retention, and eventual kidney failure.

- Regular monitoring: Routine urine and blood tests, such as serum creatinine and estimated glomerular filtration rate (eGFR), can help detect early signs of kidney damage.

- Blood pressure management: Controlling blood pressure levels is crucial in preserving kidney function.

- Medication: Certain medications, such as angiotensin-converting enzyme (ACE) inhibitors or angiotensin receptor blockers (ARBs), may be prescribed to protect kidney function.

4 . EYE COMPLICATIONS:

Diabetes can affect the eyes and increase the risk of various eye conditions, including:

- Diabetic retinopathy: High blood sugar levels damage the blood vessels in the retina, leading to vision problems, retinal detachment, and potential blindness if left untreated.

- Cataracts: Individuals with diabetes are more likely to develop cataracts, which cloud the lens of the eye and impair vision.

- Glaucoma: Diabetes increases the risk of developing glaucoma, a condition characterized by increased pressure within the eye, leading to optic nerve damage and vision loss.

Regular eye examinations, blood sugar control, blood pressure management, and early treatment interventions can help prevent or minimize the impact of these eye complications.

5 . FOOT COMPLICATIONS:

Diabetes can affect circulation and nerves in the feet, resulting in foot complications such as:

- Diabetic foot ulcers: Poor circulation and nerve damage can lead to foot sores that heal slowly and are prone to infections. In severe cases, amputation may be necessary.
- Peripheral artery disease: Reduced blood flow to the feet can cause pain, infections, and slow wound healing.

- Neuropathy: Nerve damage can cause loss of sensation, making it difficult to detect injuries or infections.

To prevent complications, it is crucial to practice regular foot care, wear proper footwear, and promptly address any concerning signs or symptoms by seeking medical attention.

6 . MENTAL HEALTH:

Diabetes management can also impact mental health and well-being. Constantly monitoring blood sugar levels, adhering to dietary restrictions, and the potential for complications may contribute to:

- Diabetes distress: The emotional burden and stress associated with managing diabetes can lead to frustration, anxiety, and depression.
- Burnout: The ongoing demands of diabetes management may result in burnout, characterized by exhaustion,

disengagement, and a decreased ability to cope effectively.

Addressing mental health concerns and seeking support from healthcare professionals, diabetes educators, counselors, or support groups is essential to promote overall well-being.

Proactive management of diabetes through regular medical check-ups, adherence to medication and treatment plans, blood sugar control, healthy lifestyle choices, and addressing risk factors is crucial in reducing the risk of complications and long-term effects. With proper care and management, individuals with diabetes can lead fulfilling

lives and minimize the impact of the disease
on their overall health.

CHAPTER 4

OVARIAN CANCER: THE WHISPERING THREAT

Ovarian cancer is a formidable illness that often goes unnoticed until its later stages, earning it the reputation of a "whispering threat." It is a type of cancer that originates in the ovaries, which are responsible for producing eggs and hormones in the female reproductive system. Ovarian cancer poses unique challenges because its early symptoms are often subtle or mistaken for less serious ailments. In this section, we will explore the nature of ovarian cancer, its risk factors, and the importance of early detection.

UNDERSTANDING OVARIAN CANCER:

Ovarian cancer occurs when abnormal cells in the ovaries multiply and form tumors. These tumors can be either benign (non-cancerous) or malignant (cancerous). Malignant ovarian tumors have the potential to invade nearby tissues and spread to other parts of the body, making them more dangerous.

SUBTLE SYMPTOMS:

Ovarian cancer is known for its lack of specific symptoms in its early stages, leading to delayed diagnosis. Common symptoms, when they do appear, may include:

- Abdominal bloating or swelling
- Pelvic pain or discomfort
- Difficulty eating or feeling full quickly
- Changes in bowel habits
- Frequent urination

Unfortunately, these symptoms are often vague and can be easily dismissed or attributed to other conditions. As a result, ovarian cancer is frequently diagnosed at advanced stages, making treatment more challenging.

RISK FACTORS:

Several factors have been associated with an increased likelihood of developing ovarian cancer:

- Age: The risk of ovarian cancer increases with age, particularly after menopause.
- Family history: Having a close relative (such as a mother, sister, or daughter) with ovarian, breast, or colorectal cancer increases the risk.
- Inherited gene mutations: Certain gene mutations, like BRCA1 and BRCA2, significantly increase the risk of developing ovarian cancer.

- Personal history of cancer: A previous diagnosis of breast, colorectal, or uterine cancer may increase the risk.

- Hormone replacement therapy: Long-term use of hormone replacement therapy after menopause may slightly increase the risk.

It is important to note that having one or more risk factors does not guarantee the development of ovarian cancer. Conversely, some women without any known risk factors may still develop the disease.

EARLY DETECTION AND PREVENTION:

Detecting ovarian cancer at an early stage is vital for improving treatment outcomes and survival rates. Unfortunately, routine screening methods for other types of cancer, such as Pap smears for cervical cancer, are not effective in detecting ovarian cancer. However, there are preventive measures and diagnostic tools available:

- Genetic counseling and testing: Women with a family history of ovarian or breast cancer may benefit from genetic testing to identify any inherited gene mutations that increase the risk.

- Pelvic exams and ultrasounds: Regular pelvic exams can help detect abnormalities, although they are not specifically designed to identify ovarian cancer. Transvaginal ultrasound may be used to visualize the ovaries and assess any suspicious findings.

- Tumor markers: Blood tests, such as CA-125 and HE4, can measure certain proteins that are often elevated in ovarian cancer. However, these markers are not definitive for diagnosing ovarian cancer and may also be elevated in non-cancerous conditions.

Maintaining a healthy lifestyle, including regular exercise, a balanced diet, and avoiding tobacco products, may help reduce the risk of ovarian cancer. Additionally, it is crucial for individuals at higher risk to consult with a healthcare professional about their specific risk factors and appropriate surveillance strategies.

Early detection and prompt medical intervention are crucial for improving the prognosis of ovarian cancer. Raising awareness among women and healthcare providers about the symptoms and risk factors can lead to earlier diagnosis and potentially save lives. If any concerning symptoms persist or if there is a family history of ovarian cancer, seeking medical attention for further evaluation is important. Remember, in the case of ovarian cancer, being aware and vigilant can make a significant difference in outcomes.

4.1 UNDERSTANDING THE COMPLEXITY AND DIFFICULTIES OF OVARIAN CANCER

Ovarian cancer is a complicated disease with unique characteristics and obstacles that make its detection and treatment particularly challenging. In this section, we will explore the nature of ovarian cancer in more depth, including its various subtypes and the specific difficulties it presents.

DIFFERENT TYPES OF OVARIAN CANCER:

Ovarian cancer consists of several subtypes, each with its own distinct features and treatment approaches. The most common types are as follows:

- Epithelial ovarian carcinoma: This form is the most prevalent, accounting for about 90% of ovarian cancer cases. It originates from the cells that line the outer surface of the ovary.
- Germ cell tumors: These tumors develop from the cells responsible for producing

eggs in the ovary. Although rare, they tend to affect younger women and have a higher likelihood of being cured.

- Stromal tumors: These tumors arise from the connective tissue cells that support the ovary. They can produce hormones and often have a favorable prognosis.

CHALLENGES IN DETECTION:

Ovarian cancer poses several challenges in terms of early detection due to its subtle symptoms and the lack of effective screening methods. Some of the key challenges include:

- Non-specific symptoms: The initial symptoms of ovarian cancer, such as abdominal bloating, pelvic pain, or changes in bowel habits, are often vague and can easily be attributed to other conditions or overlooked.

- Absence of routine screening: Unlike cervical or breast cancer, ovarian cancer does not have a standardized screening test that has proven to be highly effective. This contributes to later-stage diagnoses when the cancer has already spread beyond the ovaries.

- Silent progression: Ovarian cancer tends to spread quietly within the abdomen, with few noticeable signs until it reaches advanced stages. This makes early detection difficult, even though early detection is crucial for effective treatment.

CHALLENGES IN DIAGNOSIS:

Accurately diagnosing ovarian cancer can be challenging due to various factors:

- Lack of specific symptoms: As mentioned earlier, the symptoms of ovarian cancer are often nonspecific and resemble common gastrointestinal or gynecological issues. This can result in delayed diagnosis and treatment.

- Limitations of screening tests: The available screening tests, such as transvaginal ultrasound and tumor markers like CA-125, have limitations in terms of accuracy and specificity. False positives and false negatives can occur, leading to unnecessary investigations or missed diagnoses.

- Disease heterogeneity: Ovarian cancer is a diverse disease with different subtypes and genetic alterations, making it difficult to develop a one-size-fits-all diagnostic approach.

CHALLENGES IN TREATMENT:

Treating ovarian cancer can be complex and challenging due to various factors:

- Late-stage diagnosis: The majority of ovarian cancer cases are diagnosed at advanced stages when the cancer has spread beyond the ovaries. This requires more aggressive treatment approaches.

- Surgical complexity: Surgery plays a vital role in ovarian cancer treatment, involving the removal of the ovaries, fallopian tubes, and often other affected tissues in the abdomen. The extensive surgical procedures required can be challenging and may require the expertise of specialized gynecologic oncologists.

- Resistance to therapy: Over time, ovarian cancer has a tendency to develop resistance to chemotherapy, reducing the effectiveness of treatment. This emphasizes the need for ongoing research and the development of innovative treatment strategies.

Addressing the challenges associated with ovarian cancer requires a comprehensive approach. Increasing awareness among women and healthcare providers about the symptoms and risk factors can contribute to earlier detection. Advancements in research, including the identification of new biomarkers and targeted therapies, are crucial for improving diagnosis and treatment outcomes. Collaboration among healthcare professionals, researchers, and advocacy groups is key to overcoming the challenges posed by ovarian cancer and enhancing patient outcomes.

4.2 RISK FACTORS AND EARLY WARNING SIGNS

Understanding the factors that increase the risk and recognizing the early signs of ovarian cancer are crucial for detecting the disease early and seeking prompt medical attention. Although ovarian cancer can affect women of all ages, certain factors can elevate the risk. This section will explore the common risk factors associated with ovarian cancer and the early signs that require attention.

RISK FACTORS:

Various factors can raise a woman's risk of developing ovarian cancer:

- Age: The risk of ovarian cancer escalates with age, particularly after menopause. Most cases are diagnosed in women aged 55 and above.

- Family history: Having a close relative (such as a mother, sister, or daughter) who has had ovarian, breast, or colorectal cancer increases the risk. The risk is even higher if multiple family members are affected.

- Inherited gene mutations: Inherited gene mutations, like BRCA1 and BRCA2, significantly raise the risk of ovarian cancer. These mutations are also linked to an increased risk of breast and ovarian cancer within families.

- Personal history of cancer: A previous diagnosis of breast, colorectal, or uterine cancer may slightly increase the risk of ovarian cancer.

- Hormone-related factors: Certain hormone-related factors can influence the risk of ovarian cancer. These include early onset of menstruation, late onset of menopause, never having given birth, and the use of hormone replacement therapy (HRT) without estrogen-only formulations.

It is important to note that having one or more risk factors does not guarantee the development of ovarian cancer, and conversely, some women without any known risk factors may still develop the disease.

EARLY WARNING SIGNS:

Recognizing the early warning signs of ovarian cancer can aid in early detection. Although these signs can be subtle and resemble other conditions, they should not be disregarded. Common early warning signs of ovarian cancer include:

- Persistent abdominal bloating or swelling
- Pelvic pain or discomfort
- Difficulty eating or feeling full quickly
- Changes in bowel habits, such as constipation or diarrhea
- Frequent urination

If these symptoms occur frequently and persist for more than a few weeks, it is crucial to consult a healthcare professional for further evaluation.

SYMPTOM PATTERNS:

It is important to consider that the pattern of symptoms may be more significant than the presence of individual symptoms alone. If these warning signs are new, unusual, and occur more frequently, it is advisable to seek medical attention. Persistent and worsening symptoms that interfere with daily activities should not be ignored.

OTHER CONSIDERATIONS:

It is worth mentioning that the early warning signs of ovarian cancer are often nonspecific and can also be caused by other conditions. Therefore, a comprehensive medical evaluation is necessary to determine the underlying cause of these symptoms. If ovarian cancer is suspected, additional diagnostic tests such as imaging studies and blood tests may be recommended.

IMPORTANCE OF EARLY DETECTION:

Detecting ovarian cancer early is crucial for improving treatment outcomes and survival rates. Unfortunately, due to the absence of specific screening methods, most cases are diagnosed at advanced stages when the cancer has already spread beyond the ovaries. This poses a challenge for early detection but underscores the importance of understanding risk factors and being vigilant about warning signs.

If you have concerns about ovarian cancer or experience persistent and concerning symptoms, it is important to discuss them with a healthcare professional. They can assess your individual risk factors, perform necessary tests, and provide appropriate guidance for early detection and preventive measures.

Remember, early detection increases the chances of successful treatment and improved prognosis for ovarian cancer.

4.3 DIAGNOSIS AND TREATMENT OPTIONS

A comprehensive approach involving different medical experts and diagnostic tools is necessary to diagnose and treat ovarian cancer. In this section, we will explore the process of diagnosing ovarian cancer and discuss the available treatment choices.

DIAGNOSING OVARIAN CANCER:

When ovarian cancer is suspected based on symptoms, risk factors, or physical examination findings, the following diagnostic tests may be performed:

- Pelvic Examination: This allows healthcare providers to assess the size and shape of the ovaries and identify any abnormalities or masses.

- Imaging Tests: Procedures like transvaginal ultrasound, abdominal/pelvic CT scan, or MRI provide detailed images of the ovaries and nearby structures. These tests help determine the tumor's location, size, and spread.

- Blood Tests: Certain blood tests, such as the CA-125 test, measure the level of a protein called cancer antigen 125. Elevated levels of CA-125 may indicate ovarian cancer, although this test is not specific and can be elevated in other conditions too.

- Biopsy: A tissue sample from the ovary or a suspicious mass may be taken for analysis. A pathologist examines this sample to confirm the presence of cancer cells and determine the specific type and grade of ovarian cancer.

It is important to note that a definitive diagnosis of ovarian cancer can only be made through a biopsy and examination of the tissue sample.

STAGING OVARIAN CANCER:

Once ovarian cancer is diagnosed, it is staged to determine the extent and spread of the disease. Staging helps guide treatment decisions and prognosis. The FIGO (International Federation of Gynecology and Obstetrics) system, consisting of four stages, is commonly used for ovarian cancer:

- Stage I: The cancer is confined to the ovaries.

- Stage II: The cancer has spread to other pelvic structures, such as the fallopian tubes or uterus.

- Stage III: The cancer has spread beyond the pelvis to the abdominal lining or nearby lymph nodes.

- Stage IV: The cancer has spread to distant organs, such as the liver or lungs.

Accurate staging requires a combination of imaging tests, surgical exploration, and examination of the removed tissues.

TREATMENT OPTIONS FOR OVARIAN CANCER:

The treatment of ovarian cancer depends on factors like cancer stage, subtype, and the individual's overall health. Treatment options may include:

- Surgery: Surgery is a crucial part of ovarian cancer treatment. It involves removing the ovaries, fallopian tubes, and nearby lymph nodes. In advanced stages, it may also include the removal of the uterus and affected tissues in the abdomen.

- Chemotherapy: Anti-cancer drugs are used to destroy cancer cells in chemotherapy. It can be administered before surgery (neoadjuvant chemotherapy) to shrink the tumor or after surgery (adjuvant chemotherapy) to kill any remaining cancer cells. Chemotherapy can also be the primary treatment for advanced or recurrent ovarian cancer.

- Targeted Therapy: Targeted therapy drugs specifically interfere with molecules or pathways involved in cancer growth. They can be used in combination with chemotherapy or as maintenance therapy after initial treatment.

- Radiation Therapy: High-energy beams are used in radiation therapy to kill cancer cells. It is not commonly used as the primary treatment for ovarian cancer but may be recommended in specific situations to target particular areas.

- Hormonal Therapy: Hormonal therapy may be used for rare hormone-sensitive types of ovarian cancer, such as stromal tumors. Its goal is to block hormone effects or reduce hormone production to slow down cancer cell growth.

Treatment plans are tailored to individual circumstances based on the cancer stage, subtype, and the patient's preferences and overall health. Multidisciplinary care involving gynecologic oncologists, medical oncologists, and other specialists is essential for the best outcomes.

FOLLOW-UP CARE AND SURVEILLANCE:

After completing the initial treatment, regular follow-up visits are scheduled to monitor the patient's progress and detect any signs of recurrence. Follow-up care may include physical examinations, blood tests, and imaging studies. It is important for individuals who have had ovarian cancer to maintain open communication with their healthcare team and report any new or persistent symptoms.

CLINICAL TRIALS:

Participation in clinical trials is an important option for individuals with ovarian cancer. Clinical trials investigate new treatments, novel drug combinations, and innovative approaches to improve outcomes and quality of life for patients. By participating in clinical trials, patients can contribute to advancing ovarian cancer research and potentially access cutting-edge therapies.

Remember, each case of ovarian cancer is unique, and treatment plans are tailored to individual circumstances. It is crucial to have open and honest discussions with healthcare professionals to fully understand the available treatment options and make informed decisions.

4.4 SUPPORT AND ASSISTANCE FOR PATIENTS WITH OVARIAN CANCER

Receiving a diagnosis of ovarian cancer can be overwhelming and emotionally challenging. However, it's important to know that you're not alone on this journey. There are various services and resources in place to help you navigate the physical, emotional, and practical aspects of dealing with ovarian cancer. In this section, we will explore some of the options available to assist ovarian cancer patients and their loved ones.

SUPPORT GROUPS:

Joining support groups can provide valuable emotional support and a sense of belonging. These groups bring together individuals who are going through similar experiences, offering understanding, empathy, and encouragement. Support groups can be in-person or online, and they may be led by healthcare organizations, advocacy groups, or cancer centers.

COUNSELING AND MENTAL HEALTH SERVICES:

Dealing with ovarian cancer can have an impact on your mental and emotional well-being. Seeking professional counseling or therapy can help address feelings of anxiety, depression, or stress. Mental health professionals experienced in working with cancer patients can provide guidance, coping strategies, and emotional support to help you navigate the challenges of the disease.

EDUCATIONAL RESOURCES:

Educating yourself about ovarian cancer is crucial for understanding the disease, treatment options, and managing side effects. Many reputable organizations and websites offer reliable and up-to-date information about ovarian cancer. These resources can help answer your questions, provide guidance on self-care, and empower you to actively participate in your treatment decisions.

FERTILITY PRESERVATION:

For women of childbearing age who want to preserve their fertility, it's important to discuss fertility preservation options with healthcare providers. Ovarian cancer treatments, such as surgery and chemotherapy, can affect fertility. Fertility preservation techniques, like egg or embryo freezing, can be considered before treatment. Fertility specialists can offer guidance and explore available options.

FINANCIAL AND PRACTICAL ASSISTANCE:

Ovarian cancer treatment can pose financial and logistical challenges. There are organizations and programs that offer assistance with insurance navigation, managing medical bills, and accessing financial aid or grants. Social workers, financial counselors, and patient navigators can provide information and resources to help ease these burdens.

PALLIATIVE CARE AND HOSPICE SERVICES:

Palliative care focuses on improving the quality of life for patients with serious illnesses, including ovarian cancer. Palliative care teams provide comprehensive support, managing symptoms, and addressing physical, emotional, and spiritual needs. Hospice care, on the other hand, is specifically designed for end-of-life support, ensuring comfort and dignity for patients and their families.

ADVOCACY AND AWARENESS ORGANIZATIONS:

There are numerous organizations dedicated to ovarian cancer research, support, and raising awareness. These organizations offer a wealth of information, support networks, and community events. They also advocate for policy changes, funding for research, and improved access to care.

PERSONAL SUPPORT NETWORK:

Rely on your personal support network, including family, friends, and loved ones. Communicate your needs, share your concerns, and allow them to provide emotional support and practical assistance. Having a strong support system can make a significant difference in coping with ovarian cancer.

Remember, you're not alone on this journey. Reach out to healthcare professionals, support organizations, and trusted individuals to access the available support and resources. Each person's experience with ovarian cancer is unique, and finding the right combination of support services and resources can greatly enhance your well-being and resilience throughout the process.

CHAPTER 5

COLORECTAL CANCER: A SILENT JOURNEY TO DANGER

Colorectal cancer, a widespread and frequently undetectable illness affecting the colon and rectum, poses a significant threat. It ranks as the third most common cancer worldwide and a leading cause of cancer-related fatalities. This type of cancer usually originates from precancerous polyps, abnormal growths in the colon or rectum lining. Over time, these polyps can slowly develop into cancer, highlighting the critical importance of early detection and timely intervention for successful treatment outcomes.

THE SILENT PROGRESSION OF COLORECTAL CANCER:

Often referred to as a silent disease, colorectal cancer typically lacks noticeable symptoms in its early stages. As the tumor grows, it can obstruct the colon, leading to changes in bowel habits and symptoms such as persistent abdominal pain, rectal bleeding, or unexplained weight loss. However, these symptoms can be nonspecific and easily attributed to other conditions, resulting in the disease going unnoticed until it has advanced. This underscores the significance of regular screenings and awareness of risk factors to catch colorectal cancer in its early

stages.

RISK FACTORS ASSOCIATED WITH **COLORECTAL** Cancer:

Certain factors increase the likelihood of developing colorectal cancer, including:

- Age: The risk of colorectal cancer rises with age, with most cases occurring in individuals over the age of 50. It is recommended for individuals in this age group to undergo regular screenings.

- Family History: Having a family history of colorectal cancer or specific genetic conditions like Lynch syndrome or familial adenomatous polyposis (FAP) raises the risk. If a close relative has been diagnosed with colorectal cancer, it is important to discuss this with a healthcare provider.

- Personal History of Polyps or Inflammatory Bowel Disease: Individuals with a history of polyps in the colon or rectum, or those who have experienced inflammatory bowel disease like Crohn's disease or ulcerative colitis, face a higher risk of developing colorectal cancer.

- Lifestyle Factors: Unhealthy lifestyle choices such as a diet high in red and processed meats, low fiber intake, sedentary behavior, obesity, smoking, and excessive alcohol consumption can increase the risk of colorectal cancer.

Understanding these risk factors and discussing them with a healthcare provider is essential to determine appropriate screening and preventive measures.

SCREENING AND EARLY DETECTION:

Screening plays a vital role in the early detection and prevention of colorectal cancer. Common screening methods include:

- Colonoscopy: This procedure allows a healthcare provider to examine the entire colon and rectum using a flexible tube equipped with a camera. It enables the detection and removal of polyps, thereby reducing the risk of cancer development.

- Fecal Occult Blood Test (FOBT): This test identifies small amounts of blood in the stool, which can indicate the presence of polyps or cancer. If the test results are positive, further diagnostic tests like a colonoscopy are typically recommended.

- Flexible Sigmoidoscopy: This procedure involves examining the rectum and the lower part of the colon using a flexible tube. It can detect polyps and cancers in the lower portion of the colon.

- Stool DNA Testing: This newer screening option looks for specific DNA changes in stool samples that may indicate the presence of colorectal cancer or precancerous polyps. It is less invasive than a colonoscopy but may not be as widely available.

The choice of screening method depends on individual factors such as age, risk level, and personal preferences. Regular screenings can help identify colorectal cancer at an early stage or even before it develops, significantly enhancing treatment outcomes.

TREATMENT OPTIONS FOR COLORECTAL CANCER:

The treatment for colorectal cancer depends on the stage of the disease, tumor location, and the overall health of the individual. Common treatment options include:

- Surgery: Surgery is the primary treatment for localized colorectal cancer. It involves removing the tumor and nearby lymph nodes. In some cases, a colostomy or ileostomy may be necessary to reroute the bowel to an abdominal wall opening.

- Chemotherapy: Chemotherapy employs drugs to kill cancer cells or impede their growth. It is often used after surgery to eliminate any remaining cancer cells or in advanced stages to control the disease and improve symptoms.

- Radiation Therapy: Radiation therapy employs high-energy beams to target and destroy cancer cells. It may be used prior to surgery to shrink the tumor or after surgery to eradicate any remaining cancer cells.

- Targeted Therapy: Targeted therapy drugs specifically target certain molecules or pathways involved in cancer growth. They can be used alongside chemotherapy or as standalone treatments, depending on the specific tumor characteristics.

● Immunotherapy: Immunotherapy utilizes the body's immune system to recognize and attack cancer cells. Although currently more commonly used in other types of cancer, ongoing research on immunotherapy in colorectal cancer may establish it as a standard treatment option in the future.

The choice of treatment depends on various factors and is typically determined by a multidisciplinary team of healthcare professionals.

PREVENTION AND LIFESTYLE MODIFICATIONS:

While certain risk factors for colorectal cancer are beyond control, adopting a healthy lifestyle can significantly reduce the risk. Recommendations for prevention and minimizing the risk of colorectal cancer include:

Maintaining a balanced diet rich in fruits, vegetables, whole grains, and lean proteins, while limiting the consumption of red and processed meats.

- Regular physical activity and maintaining a healthy weight.
- Avoiding smoking and excessive alcohol consumption.
- Undergoing regular screenings as recommended by healthcare professionals based on individual risk factors.
- Managing and treating conditions such as inflammatory bowel disease or previous polyps that increase the risk of colorectal cancer.

By incorporating these preventive measures into one's lifestyle, it is possible to help decrease the risk of developing colorectal cancer and promote overall well-being.

Therefore colorectal cancer can silently progress without prominent symptoms, underscoring the significance of regular screenings, understanding risk factors, and adopting a healthy lifestyle. Early detection through screening enables timely intervention, improving treatment outcomes and survival rates. By raising awareness, promoting screening, and embracing preventive measures, we can combat this concealed journey towards danger and work towards reducing the burden of colorectal cancer.

5.1 THE STEALTHY NATURE OF COLORECTAL CANCER

Colorectal cancer is often described as a stealthy illness because it develops and advances silently, without noticeable symptoms in its early stages. This hidden characteristic presents a significant challenge in detecting the disease at an early and more treatable stage. It is essential to comprehend the stealthy attributes of colorectal cancer to raise awareness, encourage screenings, and enhance outcomes for individuals at risk.

ABSENCE OF EARLY WARNING SIGNS:

During the initial stages, colorectal cancer often does not exhibit obvious symptoms. That's why regular screenings like colonoscopies are crucial for identifying the disease before symptoms become apparent. When symptoms do arise, they can be nonspecific and easily attributed to other less concerning conditions, resulting in delayed diagnosis and treatment.

GRADUAL PROGRESSION:

Typically, colorectal cancer develops from precancerous polyps, abnormal growths in the colon or rectum. These polyps can take years to transform into cancer, providing an opportunity to detect and remove them through screening procedures. However, if left undetected or untreated, the cancer can slowly grow and spread to other body parts, posing greater challenges for treatment.

NON-SPECIFIC SYMPTOMS:

As colorectal cancer advances, it may cause symptoms such as persistent changes in bowel habits (diarrhea or constipation), rectal bleeding, abdominal pain or cramps, unexplained weight loss, fatigue, or a feeling of incomplete bowel movement. Although these symptoms may suggest colorectal cancer, they can also be associated with other gastrointestinal conditions, leading to misdiagnosis or delayed diagnosis.

IMPORTANCE OF TUMOR LOCATION:

The location of the colorectal tumor can influence the presence and severity of symptoms. Cancers in the right side of the colon tend to grow larger before causing noticeable symptoms. In contrast, tumors in the left side of the colon or rectum may trigger symptoms like rectal bleeding or changes in bowel habits at an earlier stage.

AGE AND GENETIC FACTORS:

While colorectal cancer can affect individuals of all ages, the risk increases with age, with most cases diagnosed in people over 50. Additionally, individuals with a family history of colorectal cancer or certain genetic conditions such as Lynch syndrome or familial adenomatous polyposis (FAP) face a higher risk of developing the disease.

SIGNIFICANCE OF REGULAR SCREENINGS:

Due to the stealthy nature of colorectal cancer, regular screenings play a vital role in early detection. Screening tests like colonoscopies can identify and remove precancerous polyps or detect cancer in its early stages, when treatment is more effective. The recommended age to begin screening varies based on individual risk factors, but most guidelines suggest starting at age 50 for individuals at average risk.

Increasing public awareness about the stealthy nature of colorectal cancer is essential to promote the importance of screenings, especially among high-risk individuals. By understanding the disease's silent progression and the potential absence of early warning signs, individuals can take proactive steps to prioritize their colorectal health and undergo regular screenings as advised by healthcare professionals. Through early detection, we can improve outcomes, lessen the impact of colorectal cancer, and save lives.

5.2 SCREENING AND DETECTION METHODS

Early detection and effective treatment outcomes are crucial in the screening process for colorectal cancer. There are different methods available for screening and detection, each with its own advantages and considerations. It is essential for individuals and healthcare providers to have a good understanding of these methods in order to make well-informed decisions regarding colorectal cancer screening.

COLONOSCOPY:

Colonoscopy is considered the most reliable method for screening colorectal cancer. It involves inserting a flexible tube with a camera, called a colonoscope, into the rectum to examine the entire colon. This procedure allows doctors to visually inspect the colon lining, identify and potentially remove polyps or tumors for further examination. Colonoscopy can detect both cancerous and precancerous polyps, providing diagnostic and preventive benefits. Typically performed with sedation, it is recommended every 10 years for individuals at average risk, or more frequently for those at higher risk.

MUNOCHEMICAL TEST (FIT):

FIT is a non-invasive test that detects hidden blood in the stool, which can be an indication of colorectal polyps or cancer. It involves collecting a small stool sample and sending it to a laboratory for analysis. FIT is convenient and can be done at home. It is generally recommended as an annual screening option for individuals at average risk. If the FIT result is positive, further diagnostic evaluation, such as a colonoscopy, is usually advised.

FECAL OCCULT BLOOD TEST (FOBT):

FOBT is an older stool-based screening method that detects hidden blood in the stool. Like FIT, it involves collecting a stool sample at home and sending it to a laboratory for analysis. However, FOBT is less specific than FIT and may require dietary restrictions before testing. It is recommended every one to two years for individuals at average risk. A positive FOBT result typically leads to additional diagnostic evaluation.

FLEXIBLE SIGMOIDOSCOPY:

Flexible sigmoidoscopy is a procedure that examines the rectum and the lower part of the colon using a flexible tube called a sigmoidoscope. It can help detect polyps or cancer in the lower portion of the colon. While it does not assess the entire colon like a colonoscopy, it can be a valuable screening tool, especially when combined with stool-based tests. Flexible sigmoidoscopy is generally recommended every five years.

STOOL DNA TESTING:

Stool DNA testing, also known as multi-targeted stool DNA test (MT-sDNA), is a newer screening option. It analyzes stool samples for specific DNA changes associated with colorectal cancer or precancerous polyps. The test is non-invasive and can be done at home. However, if the results are positive, a follow-up colonoscopy is required for further evaluation. Stool DNA testing may be considered every three years for individuals at average risk who prefer a non-invasive option.

VIRTUAL COLONOSCOPY (CT COLONOGRAPHY):

Virtual colonoscopy, also known as CT colonography, uses computed tomography (CT) scans to generate detailed images of the colon and rectum. It provides a comprehensive view of the colon without the need for inserting a scope. While it is less invasive than a traditional colonoscopy, it still requires bowel preparation. If polyps or abnormalities are detected, a follow-up colonoscopy is necessary. Virtual colonoscopy may be an alternative option for individuals who are unable to undergo a conventional colonoscopy.

It is important to note that the choice of screening method depends on various factors, including individual risk, preferences, and availability. It is recommended to have a discussion with a healthcare provider who can assess individual risk factors, offer guidance, and determine the most suitable screening strategy.

Regular colorectal cancer screenings are vital for early detection and prevention. By identifying precancerous polyps or detecting cancer at an early stage, screenings can significantly reduce colorectal cancer mortality rates. It is important to remember that early detection saves lives, and being proactive in colorectal cancer screening can have a substantial impact on overall health outcomes.

5.3 TREATMENT APPROACHES AND SURVIVAL RATES

The treatment of colorectal cancer depends on various factors, including the stage of the cancer, tumor location, and overall health of the patient. Treatment approaches typically involve a combination of surgery, chemotherapy, radiation therapy, targeted therapy, and immunotherapy. The goal is to eliminate or destroy cancer cells, prevent their spread, and enhance the patient's quality of life.

- Surgery is the primary treatment for localized colorectal cancer. It involves removing the tumor, along with nearby lymph nodes, and resecting the affected part of the colon or rectum. In some cases, a colostomy or ileostomy may be necessary to create an opening in the abdominal wall for waste elimination. The extent of surgery depends on the stage and location of the cancer.

- Chemotherapy uses drugs to kill or slow down cancer cells. It may be administered before surgery to shrink tumors (neoadjuvant chemotherapy) or after surgery to eliminate any remaining cancer cells (adjuvant chemotherapy). In advanced or metastatic colorectal cancer, chemotherapy may be the primary treatment option to control the disease and relieve symptoms. The specific drugs and duration of chemotherapy depend on individual factors and the stage of the cancer.

- Radiation therapy involves using high-energy beams to target and destroy cancer cells. It can be used in combination with surgery and chemotherapy, either before surgery to shrink the tumor (neoadjuvant radiation therapy) or after surgery to kill remaining cancer cells (adjuvant radiation therapy). In some cases, radiation therapy can also help alleviate symptoms such as pain or bleeding in advanced stages of colorectal cancer.

- Targeted therapy focuses on specific molecules or pathways involved in cancer growth and progression. For example, drugs like bevacizumab and cetuximab target proteins on cancer cells, inhibiting their growth and promoting their destruction. These drugs are often used in combination with chemotherapy or as standalone treatments, depending on the specific tumor characteristics and molecular markers.

- Immunotherapy works by stimulating the body's immune system to recognize and attack cancer cells. Although currently more commonly used in other cancer types, ongoing research is exploring the use of immunotherapy in colorectal cancer. Immune checkpoint inhibitors, such as pembrolizumab, are being investigated in specific cases of colorectal cancer with certain genetic features. Immunotherapy may offer new treatment options in the future.

Survival rates for colorectal cancer vary depending on factors such as the stage of the cancer at diagnosis, overall health, and treatment effectiveness. Generally, the earlier the cancer is detected and treated, the better the prognosis. According to the American Cancer Society, the five-year survival rate for localized colorectal cancer is approximately 90%, while the rate for advanced or metastatic colorectal cancer is around 14%.

It's important to note that survival rates are statistical estimates and cannot predict the outcome for an individual. Each person's experience with colorectal cancer is unique, and factors such as treatment response, overall health, and access to supportive care can influence outcomes. Close collaboration between healthcare providers and individuals affected by colorectal cancer is crucial in determining the most suitable treatment approach and providing comprehensive care throughout the treatment process.

Furthermore, advancements in treatment options, including targeted therapies and immunotherapies, continue to improve survival rates and enhance the quality of life for individuals with colorectal cancer. Ongoing research and clinical trials are focused on developing new treatments and further improving outcomes for this disease.

Remember, early diagnosis, personalized treatment approaches, and a multidisciplinary approach to care are essential factors in maximizing survival rates and ensuring the best possible outcome for individuals facing colorectal cancer.

5.4 PROMOTING AWARENESS AND PREVENTION

Raising awareness and taking preventive measures are essential for reducing the burden of colorectal cancer. Increasing knowledge and promoting early detection empower individuals to proactively prevent or identify colorectal cancer at an early and more manageable stage. The following are important aspects of promoting awareness and prevention:

EDUCATION AND INFORMATION:

Disseminating accurate and accessible information about colorectal cancer, its risk factors, and the significance of screening is crucial. Educational campaigns, public health initiatives, and healthcare providers have a vital role in delivering this information. They can highlight colorectal cancer signs and symptoms, explain screening methods, and address common misconceptions.

SCREENING GUIDELINES:

Emphasizing and encouraging adherence to colorectal cancer screening guidelines is vital. These guidelines, established by reputable organizations like the American Cancer Society, offer evidence-based recommendations on when and how often individuals should undergo screening. Healthcare providers can play a pivotal role in discussing screening options, addressing concerns, and motivating individuals to schedule regular screenings based on their risk factors.

RISK FACTOR AWARENESS:

Increasing awareness of the risk factors associated with colorectal cancer helps individuals identify their susceptibility to the disease. Age, family history, personal history of colorectal polyps, inflammatory bowel disease, and certain genetic conditions are among the factors that elevate the risk. Understanding these risk factors enables individuals to have informed discussions with healthcare providers, make necessary lifestyle changes, or undergo earlier or more frequent screenings if needed.

LIFESTYLE MODIFICATIONS:

Promoting a healthy lifestyle is a key aspect of preventing colorectal cancer. Encouraging regular physical activity, maintaining a balanced diet rich in fruits, vegetables, and whole grains, limiting processed meats and alcohol consumption, and avoiding tobacco use can reduce the risk. These lifestyle changes not only contribute to colorectal cancer prevention but also offer various other health benefits.

COMMUNITY OUTREACH AND ENGAGEMENT:

Engaging the community through outreach programs, awareness campaigns, and events helps disseminate the message of colorectal cancer prevention. Collaborating with community organizations, schools, workplaces, and healthcare providers can reach a broader audience and facilitate access to screenings and educational resources. Community engagement efforts may include informative workshops, public talks, distribution of educational materials, and partnerships with local healthcare facilities.

SURVIVOR STORIES AND SUPPORT:

Sharing stories of individuals who have successfully overcome colorectal cancer can inspire and motivate others to take preventive measures or seek timely medical attention. Survivorship programs and support groups provide platforms for affected individuals to share experiences, seek emotional support, and learn from others who have gone through similar journeys. These resources empower individuals throughout their colorectal cancer screening and treatment process.

By promoting awareness, encouraging regular screenings, and advocating for a healthy lifestyle, significant progress can be made in preventing colorectal cancer and improving outcomes for individuals at risk. Remember, early detection and prevention are crucial in reducing the impact of colorectal cancer and saving lives.

CHAPTER 6

HEPATITIS C: SILENT LIVER INVADER

Hepatitis C, often known as the "silent invader of the liver," is a viral infection primarily affecting the liver. It can go undetected for extended periods, causing gradual harm to the liver and leading to serious complications. Understanding the characteristics of hepatitis C, how it spreads, and the importance of early identification and treatment is crucial in combatting this disease, which operates silently but can be potentially deadly.

THE HEPATITIS C VIRUS:

The hepatitis C virus (HCV) is responsible for causing hepatitis C and belongs to the Flaviviridae family. The virus is mainly transmitted through contact with infected blood. Common modes of transmission include sharing needles or drug paraphernalia, receiving unscreened blood transfusions or organ transplants, or through less common routes such as needlestick injuries or sexual contact. Although less common, transmission from mother to child during childbirth is also possible.

THE SILENT NATURE OF HEPATITIS C:

Hepatitis C is often described as a "silent" disease because it can remain asymptomatic for many years or even decades. Many individuals infected with HCV are unaware of their infection until significant liver damage occurs or until routine blood tests reveal abnormal liver function. This silent progression underscores the importance of early detection and treatment to prevent long-term complications.

LONG-TERM EFFECTS AND COMPLICATIONS:

If left untreated, chronic hepatitis C infection can lead to severe liver damage, including liver cirrhosis, liver failure, and hepatocellular carcinoma (liver cancer). These complications may develop over several decades, and the risk increases with the duration of the infection. It is crucial to identify and treat hepatitis C early to prevent irreversible liver damage.

DIAGNOSIS AND TESTING:

Hepatitis C can be diagnosed through blood tests that detect the presence of HCV antibodies or viral genetic material (RNA). Testing is recommended for individuals at an increased risk, including those with a history of injection drug use, previous blood transfusions, or known exposure to infected blood. Additionally, screening is recommended for all individuals born between 1945 and 1965, as this population has a higher prevalence of hepatitis C.

TREATMENT OPTIONS:

Fortunately, medical advancements have led to highly effective treatments for hepatitis C. Antiviral medications, known as direct-acting antivirals (DAAs), have revolutionized the treatment landscape. These medications can cure hepatitis C in the majority of cases, with cure rates exceeding 95%. Treatment duration and specific medications depend on various factors, including the HCV genotype, the presence of liver damage, and individual patient characteristics.

PREVENTION AND RISK REDUCTION:

Preventing hepatitis C primarily involves avoiding exposure to infected blood. This includes practicing safe injection practices, using sterile needles and equipment, and avoiding the sharing of personal hygiene items such as razors or toothbrushes. Screening of blood products and organ donations has significantly reduced the risk of acquiring hepatitis C through blood transfusions or transplants. Education on safe sexual practices and the use of barrier methods, such as condoms, can also reduce the risk of transmission.

PUBLIC HEALTH EFFORTS AND AWARENESS:

Public health initiatives and awareness campaigns play a crucial role in combating hepatitis C. These efforts aim to raise awareness about the disease, promote testing among at-risk populations, and facilitate access to care and treatment. Vaccination against hepatitis B, another viral infection that can cause liver disease, is also essential, as individuals with both hepatitis B and hepatitis C infections are at increased risk of liver damage.

SUPPORT AND CARE:

Living with hepatitis C can be emotionally and physically challenging. Supportive care and access to appropriate healthcare resources are essential for individuals living with the disease. Support groups, patient education programs, and counseling services can provide emotional support, while healthcare providers can offer guidance on managing the disease, coping with side effects of treatment, and making necessary lifestyle modifications.

In conclusion, hepatitis C is an insidious invader of the liver that can cause severe liver damage if left untreated. Early detection through testing and access to effective antiviral treatment are critical in preventing long-term complications and improving overall outcomes for individuals with hepatitis C. Promoting awareness, practicing risk reduction strategies, and providing support to those affected by the disease are vital components in the fight against hepatitis C.

6.1 UNVEILING HEPATITIS C: CAUSES AND TRANSMISSION

Hepatitis C, a disease primarily affecting the liver, is caused by the hepatitis C virus (HCV). Understanding how it is contracted and transmitted is vital for preventing its dissemination and reducing the burden it places on individuals. Let's delve into the fundamental aspects of hepatitis C, including its causes and modes of transmission:

THE HEPATITIS C VIRUS (HCV):

HCV is a member of the Flaviviridae family and is primarily transmitted through contact with infected blood. It is considered a bloodborne virus, capable of surviving for a limited time outside the body, which allows for transmission through various means.

TRANSMISSION MODES:

a. Injection Drug Use: Sharing needles, syringes, or other drug paraphernalia is a significant risk factor for contracting hepatitis C. Even the tiniest amounts of blood containing HCV can be transferred when drug equipment is shared.

b. Blood Transfusions and Organ Transplants: Before the implementation of widespread screening for blood and organ donations, HCV transmission through these procedures was common. However, rigorous screening measures have significantly reduced the risk of acquiring hepatitis C in this manner.

c. Healthcare-Related Exposures: Accidental exposures to contaminated needles or medical equipment, such as needlestick injuries, pose a potential risk for hepatitis C transmission. This risk primarily applies to healthcare workers who come into contact with blood or sharp instruments.

d. Mother-to-Child Transmission: Although relatively uncommon, pregnant women with hepatitis C can transmit the virus to their babies during childbirth. The risk of transmission is higher if the mother has a high viral load or is co-infected with HIV.

e. Sexual Transmission: While sexual transmission of hepatitis C is possible, it is considered less frequent than other modes of transmission. The risk increases during unprotected sexual intercourse, particularly when blood-to-blood contact occurs, such as during rough or traumatic sexual practices.

f. Other Risk Factors: Sharing personal hygiene items, such as razors or toothbrushes, which may have come into contact with infected blood, can also pose a less common mode of hepatitis C transmission.

LOW-RISK TRANSMISSION ROUTES:

Unlike some other viral infections like hepatitis B, casual contact such as hugging, kissing, or sharing food or drinks does not readily transmit hepatitis C. It is also not transmitted through respiratory droplets or breastfeeding, unless the nipple is cracked and bleeding. Nonetheless, it is important to exercise caution and take appropriate preventive measures to minimize the risk of transmission.

PREVENTION:

Preventing the transmission of hepatitis C involves adopting various strategies:

a. Safe Injection Practices: Individuals who inject drugs should never share needles, syringes, or other equipment. Access to sterile needles and drug paraphernalia through programs like needle exchange programs or syringe service programs can help reduce the risk of hepatitis C transmission.

b. Screening of Blood and Organ Donations: Thorough screening procedures for donated blood and organs have significantly decreased the risk of acquiring hepatitis C through transfusions or transplants. These measures ensure that only safe and HCV-free blood and organs are used for medical procedures.

c. Safer Sexual Practices: While the risk of sexual transmission of hepatitis C is relatively low, practicing safe sex by using barrier methods, such as condoms, can further reduce the risk of transmission. It is particularly important to use protection during sexual activities that involve the potential for blood-to-blood contact.

d. Harm Reduction Programs: Engaging in harm reduction programs, such as substance abuse treatment, counseling, and support services, can help individuals lower their risk of hepatitis C transmission by addressing underlying factors contributing to high-risk behaviors.

e. Education and Awareness: Promoting education and raising awareness about hepatitis C transmission, risk factors, and preventive measures is crucial. Public health campaigns, healthcare provider education, and community outreach efforts play a pivotal role in disseminating accurate information and dispelling misconceptions surrounding the disease.

By comprehending the causes and modes of transmission of hepatitis C, individuals can take proactive steps to prevent its spread. Implementing safe injection practices, advocating for comprehensive screening procedures, promoting safer sexual practices, and increasing education and awareness are key strategies in minimizing the impact of hepatitis C and safeguarding individuals from contracting the virus.

6.2 DETECTING HEPATITIS C: TESTING AND DIAGNOSIS

Detecting hepatitis C in a timely manner and diagnosing the infection are vital in preventing disease progression, reducing complications, and initiating suitable treatment. Hepatitis C testing involves specific laboratory procedures aimed at identifying the presence of the virus or antibodies against it. Here are the key aspects of hepatitis C testing and diagnosis:

SCREENING RECOMMENDATIONS:

Various organizations, including the Centers for Disease Control and Prevention (CDC) and the World Health Organization (WHO), have established guidelines to identify individuals at risk of hepatitis C infection. These guidelines typically recommend screening for individuals with specific risk factors, such as current or past injection drug use, history of receiving unscreened blood transfusions or organ transplants, long-term hemodialysis treatment, HIV infection, being born to a mother with hepatitis C, healthcare workers after needlestick injuries or accidental exposures, and individuals with signs or symptoms of liver disease. Additionally, some guidelines recommend one-time screening for all individuals born between 1945 and 1965, as this population has a higher prevalence of hepatitis C.

ANTIBODY TESTING:

The initial screening test for hepatitis C usually involves an antibody test. This test detects the presence of antibodies produced by the immune system in response to HCV infection. A positive antibody test indicates past or current infection, but it does not necessarily confirm ongoing viral replication.

NUCLEIC ACID TESTING (NAT):

If the antibody test is positive, confirmatory testing using nucleic acid testing (NAT) is conducted. NAT identifies the presence of viral genetic material (HCV RNA) in the blood, indicating active viral replication. It confirms the presence of an ongoing hepatitis C infection.

GENOTYPE TESTING:

After confirming a hepatitis C infection, additional testing may be performed to determine the specific HCV genotype. Hepatitis C has multiple genotypes and subtypes, which can influence treatment decisions and outcomes. Genotype testing helps tailor the most appropriate antiviral treatment regimen.

LIVER FUNCTION TESTS:

Liver function tests are commonly performed as part of the diagnostic process.

These tests measure various enzymes and proteins released by the liver. Elevated levels of liver enzymes, such as alanine transaminase (ALT) and aspartate transaminase (AST), indicate liver inflammation and potential damage.

FIBROSIS ASSESSMENT:

In certain cases, additional tests may be conducted to assess the extent of liver fibrosis (scarring) caused by hepatitis C. These tests, like transient elastography or liver biopsy, aid in determining the level of liver damage and guide treatment decisions.

RETESTING AND MONITORING:

For individuals who test negative for hepatitis C but are considered at ongoing risk of infection, regular retesting may be recommended. Monitoring liver function tests and assessing liver health through periodic screenings are also crucial for individuals with chronic hepatitis C infection.

CONFIDENTIALITY AND SUPPORT:

Maintaining confidentiality and providing support throughout the testing and diagnosis process is essential. Healthcare providers should offer counseling, education, and emotional support to individuals undergoing hepatitis C testing. This includes discussing the implications of test results, explaining available treatment options, addressing concerns, and providing resources for further information or support.

Detecting and diagnosing hepatitis C early enables timely intervention, appropriate treatment, and monitoring of liver health. Screening guidelines, antibody testing, confirmatory testing, genotyping, liver function tests, and fibrosis assessments collectively contribute to a comprehensive diagnostic approach. Through effective testing and diagnosis, individuals can receive the necessary care and support to manage hepatitis C and minimize its impact on liver health.

6.3 TREATMENT OPTIONS AND MANAGEMENT STRATEGIES

Successful management strategies and effective treatment options are crucial in the fight against hepatitis C and the prevention of its long-term complications. The primary objective of treatment is to attain a sustained virologic response (SVR), which involves eliminating the virus from the body and preventing its replication. Let's explore the available treatment options and strategies for managing hepatitis C:

ANTIVIRAL MEDICATIONS:

Recent advances in hepatitis C treatment have introduced direct-acting antiviral (DAA) medications, which have revolutionized the field. These medications specifically target various stages of the hepatitis C virus (HCV) replication cycle, inhibiting viral replication and allowing the immune system to clear the virus. DAAs are highly effective, with cure rates exceeding 95% for most genotypes. Treatment duration typically lasts between 8 to 12 weeks, depending on the genotype and individual factors.

Individualized Treatment Approach:

The treatment for hepatitis C is tailored to each individual based on several factors, including the HCV genotype, the presence of liver fibrosis or cirrhosis, concurrent medical conditions, and past treatment history. Healthcare providers evaluate these factors to determine the most appropriate antiviral medication regimen and treatment duration for each patient.

MONITORING AND FOLLOW-UP:

Regular monitoring is essential during and after treatment to assess treatment response and ensure patient safety. This involves conducting liver function tests, checking HCV RNA levels, and possibly monitoring other laboratory markers. Close follow-up enables healthcare providers to evaluate treatment effectiveness, identify potential side effects, and make adjustments to the treatment plan if necessary.

LIFESTYLE MODIFICATIONS:

Implementing certain lifestyle modifications can support the management of hepatitis C and overall liver health. These modifications may include:

- Abstaining from alcohol: Alcohol can exacerbate liver damage and interfere with the effectiveness of antiviral treatment. It is crucial to refrain from consuming alcohol to alleviate strain on the liver.

- Adopting a balanced diet: A healthy diet promotes liver function and overall well-being. It is recommended to consume a diverse range of nutrient-rich foods, such as fruits, vegetables, whole grains, and lean proteins. Individuals with advanced liver disease may require tailored dietary modifications based on their specific needs.

- Engaging in exercise and physical activity: Regular exercise aids in maintaining overall health, improving liver function, and reducing the risk of complications associated with hepatitis C. It is important to consult healthcare providers before initiating an exercise program, especially for individuals with advanced liver disease.

- Avoiding hepatotoxic medications: Certain medications, including nonsteroidal anti-inflammatory drugs (NSAIDs) and some herbal supplements, can cause liver damage or interfere with antiviral treatment. It is crucial to consult healthcare providers before taking any medications or supplements to ensure their safety.

VACCINATION:

Individuals with chronic hepatitis C infection, who are not immune to hepatitis A or hepatitis B, are recommended to receive vaccinations against these viruses. Contracting hepatitis A or hepatitis B in addition to hepatitis C can result in further liver damage and complicate the management of hepatitis C.

EMOTIONAL AND PSYCHOSOCIAL SUPPORT:

Living with hepatitis C can have emotional and psychological impacts. It is important for individuals to have access to supportive resources, such as counseling, support groups, and educational materials. These resources can help individuals cope with the emotional challenges associated with the diagnosis, treatment, and long-term management of hepatitis C.

REGULAR LIVER HEALTH MONITORING:

Even after achieving SVR through successful treatment, regular monitoring of liver health remains important. This involves periodic liver function tests, imaging studies, and assessments for the development of liver-related complications, such as cirrhosis or hepatocellular carcinoma. Long-term follow-up allows healthcare providers to intervene early if any liver-related issues arise.

By employing effective treatment options, individualized approaches, and comprehensive management strategies, individuals living with hepatitis C can find hope. Antiviral medications, lifestyle modifications, monitoring, vaccination, and emotional support are integral components of managing the disease and improving long-term outcomes. With proper care and management, individuals can lead healthy lives and reduce the risk of complications associated with hepatitis C.

6.4 EDUCATION AND PREVENTION EFFORTS

Education and prevention efforts are crucial for decreasing the impact of hepatitis C by enhancing awareness, advocating for prevention methods, and empowering individuals to take proactive measures. The following are key elements of education and prevention initiatives for hepatitis C:

RAISING PUBLIC AWARENESS:

Public health organizations, healthcare providers, and community groups play a pivotal role in conducting campaigns to educate the general population about hepatitis C. These campaigns aim to enhance understanding of risk factors, modes of transmission, and the importance of testing and treatment.

TARGETED EDUCATION:

Tailored education efforts focus on populations at higher risk of hepatitis C, such as individuals who inject drugs, people with a history of blood transfusions or organ transplants before widespread screening, and those living with HIV. Providing specific information about risk reduction strategies, testing, and treatment options is vital to effectively reach these populations.

HEALTHCARE PROVIDER TRAINING:

Healthcare providers play a critical role in identifying and managing hepatitis C. It is crucial to ensure that they receive adequate training and education on the latest guidelines, testing protocols, treatment options, and counseling techniques. This equips them to provide accurate information and deliver quality care to patients.

SCREENING AND TESTING PROGRAMS:

Implementing screening and testing programs in high-risk settings, including substance abuse treatment centers, prisons, and community health clinics, can help identify individuals with undiagnosed hepatitis C. These programs should incorporate accessible and confidential testing services, linkage to care, and follow-up support.

HARM REDUCTION PROGRAMS:

Harm reduction programs, such as needle exchange programs and syringe service programs, are pivotal in preventing hepatitis C transmission among people who inject drugs. These programs provide sterile needles and syringes, educate individuals on safer injection practices, offer overdose prevention measures, and provide access to substance abuse treatment and support services.

PREVENTION STRATEGIES:

Promoting preventive measures is vital in reducing the spread of hepatitis C. Key prevention strategies include:

- Safe Injection Practices: Encouraging individuals who inject drugs to use sterile needles, syringes, and other equipment, and to never share them.

- Safer Sexual Practices: Promoting the use of barrier methods, such as condoms, during sexual activity to reduce the risk of sexual transmission.

- Blood and Organ Donation Safety: Ensuring rigorous screening procedures for donated blood and organs to minimize the risk of hepatitis C transmission through transfusions and transplants.

- Mother-to-Child Transmission Prevention: Implementing measures to prevent mother-to-child transmission, such as screening pregnant women for hepatitis C and providing appropriate interventions during pregnancy and childbirth.

- Standard Precautions in Healthcare Settings: Promoting adherence to standard precautions, including proper infection control practices, to prevent healthcare-related exposures to hepatitis C.

COLLABORATION AND PARTNERSHIPS:

Collaborative efforts between public health agencies, healthcare providers, community organizations, and advocacy groups are crucial for implementing comprehensive education and prevention programs. These partnerships help leverage resources, share expertise, and reach diverse populations with targeted messages and interventions.

ACCESS TO TESTING AND TREATMENT:

Ensuring affordable and accessible testing and treatment options is essential for individuals at risk of or living with hepatitis C. This involves addressing barriers such as cost, healthcare disparities, and limited access to healthcare services.

By prioritizing education, prevention strategies, and collaborative efforts, it is possible to reduce the incidence and impact of hepatitis C. Continued advocacy, public awareness campaigns, targeted education programs, and comprehensive prevention initiatives are key to achieving the goal of eliminating hepatitis C as a public health threat.

CONCLUSION

EMPOWERING ACTION AGAINST SILENT KILLERSA

Diseases like hypertension, diabetes, ovarian cancer, colorectal cancer, and hepatitis C are often referred to as silent killers because they pose serious threats to our health and well-being without showing noticeable symptoms until they reach advanced stages. Detecting and preventing these diseases early on is crucial.

Understanding the concept of silent killers highlights the importance of taking proactive measures. By raising awareness and promoting regular screenings, we can identify these diseases at an early stage when interventions are most effective. Timely detection enables prompt medical intervention, leading to better treatment outcomes and an improved quality of life.

Prevention strategies play a significant role in combating silent killers. Making lifestyle changes such as adopting a healthy diet, engaging in regular physical activity, avoiding tobacco, and managing stress can greatly reduce the risk of developing these diseases. Additionally, targeted prevention efforts such as vaccination programs and initiatives to minimize the spread of infectious diseases are important.

Having comprehensive treatment options and management strategies is equally important. Medical advancements have provided effective medications and interventions for managing these diseases. Timely diagnosis, appropriate treatment, and adherence to prescribed regimens are crucial in mitigating long-term effects and complications associated with these conditions.

Empowering individuals with knowledge and resources is a key aspect of fighting silent killers. Educational campaigns, healthcare provider training, and community outreach programs help spread accurate information, encourage healthy behaviors, and promote early intervention. By increasing public awareness, ensuring access to healthcare services, and fostering collaboration, individuals can take control of their health and make informed decisions.

Support networks and resources are vital for individuals living with these conditions. Emotional and psychosocial support, counseling, and patient advocacy groups provide invaluable assistance in addressing the challenges faced by patients and their families. Encouraging open dialogue, sharing personal experiences, and promoting empathy create a supportive environment where individuals feel empowered and understood.

In conclusion, the concept of silent killers emphasizes the importance of vigilance, early detection, prevention, and treatment. Through education, prevention efforts, and support systems, we can collectively combat these diseases and improve health outcomes for individuals and communities. Taking comprehensive action against silent killers requires raising awareness, prevention, access to care, and a supportive environment. Together, we can make a significant impact in the fight against these silent yet dangerous adversaries.